ABC
Arteri

Third Edition

BMA

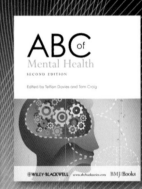
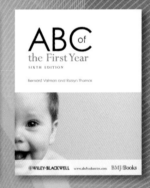
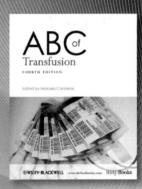
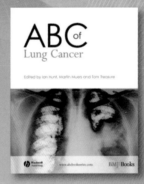
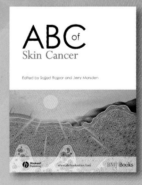
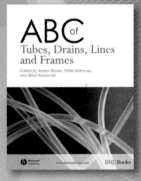

ABC of

Arterial and Venous Disease

Third Edition

EDITED BY

Tim England

Honorary Consultant Stroke Physician & Clinical Associate Professor
Division of Medical Sciences & Graduate Entry Medicine
School of Medicine, Faculty of Medicine & Health Sciences
University of Nottingham
Royal Derby Hospital Centre
Derby, UK

Akhtar Nasim

Consultant Vascular Surgeon & Honorary Senior Lecturer
Department of Vascular & Endovascular Surgery
Leicester Royal Infirmary
Leicester, UK

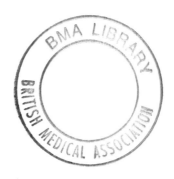

WILEY Blackwell

BMJ Books

Library of Congress Cataloging-in-Publication Data

ABC of arterial and venous disease / edited by Tim England and Akhtar Nasim. – Third edition.

   p. ; cm. – (ABC series)

Includes bibliographical references and index.

ISBN 978-1-118-74068-2 (paper)

I. England, Tim (Timothy J.), 1978- editor. II. Nasim, Akhtar, 1966- editor. III. Series: ABC series (Malden, Mass.)

[DNLM: 1. Vascular Diseases – diagnosis. 2. Vascular Diseases – therapy. WG 500]

RC691

616.1′3 – dc23

2014020542

A catalogue record for this book is available from the British Library.

Contents

Preface

Globally, the consequences of vascular disease on health have reached epidemic proportions and there is a need for continual evaluation of new therapies to reduce this significant burden on both the individual and the society.

Potential pathophysiological mechanisms affecting blood vessels are multiple, including atherosclerosis and systemic inflammation, that lead to vessel occlusion, embolism, aneurysm formation or rupture. There is consequential dysfunction or loss of tissue viability distal to a lesion, potentially leading to symptoms in any vascular bed.

Since publication of the second edition in 2009, there have been important advances in the way we approach and treat arterial and venous disease, for example, the wider introduction of novel orally active anticoagulants to prevent or treat venous and arterial thrombosis. Hence, with contributions from leading physicians, surgeons and radiologists, this new edition aims to summarise how we assess and treat the multitude of presentations of vascular disease.

Further to updates from the second edition, we have provided additional chapters on coronary heart disease, mesenteric ischaemia and arteriovenous malformations (AVM). The book is aimed at the non-specialist, and where possible, we have provided current clinical guidelines. Moreover, a clinical case vignette has been included where appropriate to provide real-life examples of current specialist practice. We hope the book is informative and interesting while providing up-to-date material on best practice of evidence-based medicine.

Tim England
Akhtar Nasim
April 2014

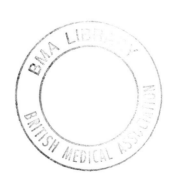

Contributors

William D. Adair
Consultant Radiologist, Leicester Royal Infirmary, UK

David Adlam
Senior Lecturer and Consultant Cardiologist,
Department of Cardiovascular Sciences, University of Leicester, UK

Asif Adnan
Specialty Registrar and Fellow in Interventional Cardiology,
Royal Derby Hospital, UK

Nishath Altaf
Clinical Lecturer in Vascular Surgery, School of Medicine, University of
Nottingham, UK

Daryll Baker
Consultant Vascular Surgeon, Royal Free Hospital, London, UK

Matthew J. Bown
Senior Lecturer, Department of Cardiovascular Sciences, University of
Leicester, UK

Nikesh Dattani
Clinical Research Fellow, Department of Cardiovascular Sciences, University
of Leicester, UK

Huw O.B. Davies
Specialist Registrar in Vascular Surgery, Heart of England NHS FT,
Birmingham, UK

Robert S.M. Davies
Consultant Vascular & Endovascular Surgeon, Department of Vascular and
Endovascular Surgery, Leicester Royal Infirmary, UK

Richard Donnelly
Professor of Vascular Medicine, Division of Medical Sciences & GEM, School
of Medicine, University of Nottingham, UK

Ruth A. England
Consultant in Palliative Medicine, Royal Derby Hospital, UK

Timothy J. England
Clinical Associate Professor & Honorary Consultant Stroke Physician,
Division of Medical Sciences & GEM, School of Medicine, University of
Nottingham, UK

Thomas E. Kalogirou
Senior Vascular Surgery Trainee,
5th Department of Surgery, Medical School, Aristotle University of
Thessaloniki, Hippocratio Hospital, Greece

Christos D. Karkos
Consultant Vascular Surgeon & Senior Lecturer,
5th Department of Surgery, Medical School, Aristotle University of
Thessaloniki, Hippocratio Hospital, Greece

Vaughan L. Keeley
Consultant in Palliative Medicine,
Royal Derby Hospital, UK

Janson C.H. Leung
Consultant Renal Physician, Royal Derby Hospital, UK

Shane MacSweeney
Consultant Vascular Surgeon,
Queen's Medical Centre, Nottingham, UK

Mark J. McCarthy
Consultant Vascular & Endovascular Surgeon, Department of Vascular and
Endovascular Surgery, Leicester Royal Infirmary, UK

Greg S. McMahon
Specialist Registrar in Vascular Surgery, Leicester Royal Infirmary, UK

Matthew D. Morgan
Clinical Senior Lecturer in Renal Medicine, School of Immunity and
Infection, College of Medical & Dental Sciences, University of
Birmingham, UK

Akhtar Nasim
Consultant Vascular & Endovascular Surgeon, Leicester Royal Infirmary, UK

Mario De Nunzio
Consultant Radiologist, Royal Derby Hospital, UK

Sue Pavord
Consultant Haematologist, University Hospitals of Leicester
NHS Trust, UK

Harjeet Rayt
Specialist Registrar in Vascular Surgery, Leicester Royal Infirmary, UK

J. Mark Scriven

Consultant Vascular Surgeon, Heart of England NHS FT, Birmingham, UK

David A. Sidloff

Clinical Research Fellow, Department of Cardiovascular Sciences, University of Leicester, UK

Stuart W. Smith

Clinical Lecturer in Renal Medicine, School of Immunity and Infection, College of Medical & Dental Sciences, University of Birmingham, UK

E. Kate Waters

Specialist Registrar in Radiology, Leicester Royal Infirmary, UK

Amy Webster

Specialist Registrar in Haematology, University Hospitals of Leicester NHS Trust, UK

CHAPTER 1

Pathogenesis of Atherosclerosis and Methods of Arterial and Venous Assessment

Mario De Nunzio[1] and Timothy J. England[2]

[1] Derby Hospitals NHS Foundation Trust, Royal Derby Hospital, UK
[2] Division of Medical Sciences & GEM, School of Medicine, University of Nottingham, UK

OVERVIEW

- Atherosclerosis is a chronic inflammatory disorder
- The ankle–brachial pressure index (ABPI), calculated from the ratio of ankle systolic blood pressure (SBP) to brachial SBP, is a sensitive marker of arterial insufficiency in the lower limb
- Blood velocity increases through an area of narrowing. Typically, a 2-fold increase in peak systolic velocity compared with the velocity in a proximal adjacent segment of the same artery usually signifies a stenosis of 50% or more
- In detecting femoral and popliteal artery disease, duplex ultrasonography has a sensitivity of 80% and a specificity of 90–100%
- The introduction of multidetector computed tomography (MDCT) has had a dramatic effect on vascular imaging. Computed tomography pulmonary angiography (CTPA) for suspected pulmonary embolism (PE) is a good example, but computed tomography angiography (CTA) and magnetic resonance angiography (MRA) are widely used to investigate large artery pathology
- Colour duplex scanning is both sensitive and specific (90–100% in most series) for detecting proximal deep vein thrombosis (DVT).

Pathogenesis of atherosclerosis

Atherosclerosis is a chronic inflammatory disorder that results in hardening and thickening of arterial walls. Although it inevitably accompanies aging, it is not a degenerative process. The initial insult, called a 'fatty streak', is a purely inflammatory lesion and has been observed in infants. Over many years, circulating monocyte-derived macrophages adhere to and invade the arterial wall. An inflammatory response, proliferation of vascular smooth muscle cells and deposition of cholesterol and other lipids create arterial plaques. The insult creates a prothrombotic environment and induces the release of inflammatory mediators including cytokines, growth factors and hydrolytic enzymes. Over time, the plaques narrow the arterial lumen (and at times dilate it) and subsequently rupture, causing platelet activation, aggregation and resultant thrombus and embolus formation (Figure 1.1). It remains unclear as to what causes a stable plaque to rupture but it may be due to mechanical stress (e.g. hypertension) and the large lipid core redistributing shear stress over weakened areas of a thin fibrous cap.

It is recognised that increasing age, a genetic predisposition, male sex, hypertension, lipid abnormalities (in particular, LDL-cholesterol), diabetes, chronic high alcohol intake and cigarette smoking (causing an increase in free radicals) increase the risk of atherogenesis and endothelial dysfunction. Atherosclerosis mainly affects large and medium-sized arteries at places of arterial branching (e.g. carotid bifurcation). Symptoms occur when there is insufficient blood flow to the vascular bed as a result of

1 *in situ* thrombotic arterial occlusion,
2 low flow distal to an occluded or severely narrowed artery or
3 embolism from an atherosclerotic plaque or thrombus.

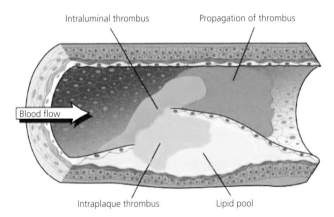

Figure 1.1 Spontaneous rupture or fissuring of an atherosclerotic plaque exposes the lipid-rich core and triggers platelet activation and platelet aggregation. The platelet GP IIb/IIIa receptor activation binds fibrinogen and leads to intravascular thrombus formation, resulting in complete or near-complete vessel occlusion. Clinically, this often presents with a life-threatening unstable event such as an acute coronary syndrome, acute limb ischaemia or stroke.

ABC of Arterial and Venous Disease, Third Edition.
Edited by Tim England and Akhtar Nasim.
© 2015 John Wiley & Sons, Ltd. Published 2015 by John Wiley & Sons, Ltd.

Clots occurring in the venous system are often evaluated referencing the principles of Virchow's triad, the three broad categories that contribute to thrombosis: venous stasis due to prolonged immobility, endothelial and vessel wall injury, for example, due to radiation or medical devices, and hypercoagulability states such as patients with malignancy or clotting factor deficiency.

Investigating vascular disease

Diagnostic and therapeutic decisions in patients with vascular disease are guided primarily by the history and physical examination. However, the accuracy and accessibility of non-invasive investigations have greatly increased due to technological advances in computed tomography (CT) and magnetic resonance (MR) scanning. Computed tomography angiography (CTA) and magnetic resonance angiography (MRA) continue to evolve rapidly and are best described as 'minimally invasive' techniques when used with intravenous (i.v.) contrast. This chapter describes the main investigative techniques used in arterial and venous diseases.

Principles of vascular ultrasound

In its simplest form, ultrasound is transmitted as a continuous beam from a probe that contains two piezoelectric crystals. The transmitting crystal produces ultrasound at a fixed frequency (set by the operator according to the depth of the vessel being examined), while the receiving crystal vibrates in response to reflected waves and produces an output voltage. Conventional B-mode (brightness mode) ultrasonography records the ultrasound waves reflected from tissue interfaces and a two-dimensional picture is built according to the reflective properties of the tissues.

Ultrasound signals reflected off stationary surfaces have the same frequency with which they were transmitted, but the principle underlying Doppler ultrasonography is that signals reflected from moving objects, e.g. red blood cells, undergo a frequency shift in proportion to the velocity of the target. The output from a continuous-wave Doppler ultrasound is most frequently presented as an audible signal (e.g. a hand-held pencil Doppler, Figure 1.2), so that a sound is heard whenever there is movement of blood in the vessel being examined. With continuous-wave ultrasonography, there is little scope for restricting the area of tissue that is being examined because any sound waves that are intercepted by the receiving crystal will produce an output signal. The solution is to use pulsed ultrasound. This enables the investigator to focus on a specific tissue plane by transmitting a pulse of ultrasound and closing the receiver except when signals from a predetermined depth are returning. For example, the centre of an artery and the areas close to the vessel wall can be examined in turn.

Examination of an arterial stenosis shows an increase in blood velocity through the area of narrowing. The site(s) of any stenotic lesions can be identified by serial placement of the Doppler probe along the extremities. Criteria to define a stenosis vary between laboratories, but a 2-fold increase in peak systolic velocity compared with the velocity in a proximal adjacent segment of the artery usually signifies a stenosis of ≥50% (Table 1.1). The normal (triphasic)

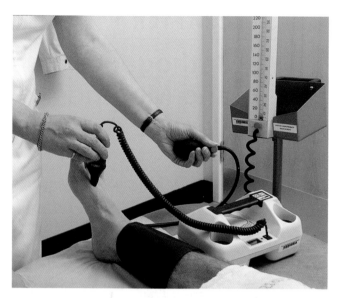

Figure 1.2 A hand-held pencil Doppler being used to measure the ankle–brachial pressure index.

Table 1.1 Relationship between increased blood velocity and degree of stenosis.

Diameter of stenosis (%)	Peak systolic velocity (m/s)*	Peak diastolic velocity (m/s)*	Internal carotid: common carotid artery ratio†
0–39	<1.1	<0.45	<1.8
4–59	1.1–1.49	<0.45	<1.8
60–79	1.5–2.49	0.45–1.4	1.8–3.7
80–99	2.5–6.1	>1.4	>3.7
>99 (critical)	Very low	NA	NA

*Measured in the lower part of the internal carotid artery.
†Ratio of peak systolic velocity in internal carotid artery stenosis relative to the velocity in the proximal common carotid artery.

Doppler velocity waveform is made up of three components that correspond to different phases of arterial flow (Figure 1.3):

- Rapid antegrade flow reaching a peak during systole
- Transient reversal of flow during early diastole
- Slow antegrade flow during late diastole.

Doppler examination of an artery distal to a stenosis shows characteristic changes in the velocity profile (Figure 1.3d):

- The rate of rise is delayed and the amplitude decreased
- The transient flow reversal in early diastole is lost
- In severe disease conditions, the Doppler waveform flattens; in critical limb ischaemia, it may be undetectable.

Investigations of arterial disease

Ankle–brachial pressure index

Under normal conditions, systolic blood pressure (SBP) in the legs is equal to or slightly greater than the SBP in the upper limbs. In the presence of an arterial stenosis, a reduction in pressure occurs

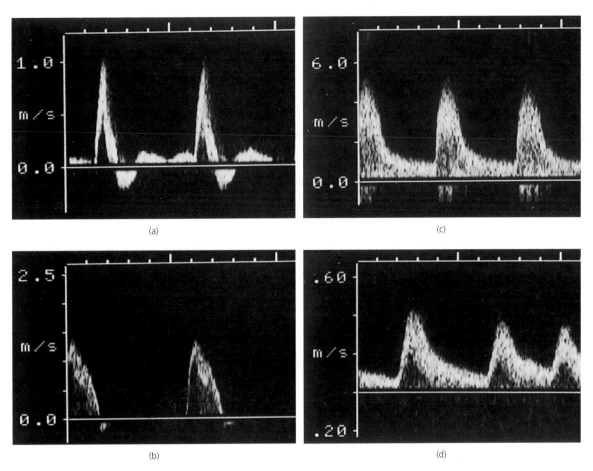

(a)

(c)

(b)

(d)

Figure 1.3 Doppler velocity waveforms: (a) a triphasic waveform in a normal artery; (b) a biphasic waveform, with increased velocity, through a mild stenosis; (c) a monophasic waveform, with a marked increase in velocity, through a tight stenosis; and (d) a dampened monophasic waveform, with reduced velocity, recorded distal to a tight stenosis.

distal to the lesion. The ankle–brachial pressure index (ABPI), calculated from the ratio of ankle SBP to brachial SBP, is a sensitive marker of arterial insufficiency in the lower limb. The highest pressure measured in any ankle artery is used as the numerator in the calculation of the ABPI. An ABPI of ≥1.0 is normal and a value <0.9 is abnormal. Patients with claudication tend to have ABPIs in the range 0.5–0.9, while those with critical ischaemia usually have an index of <0.5. In patients with diabetes (in whom distal vessels are often calcified and incompressible), SBP measured in the lower limbs may be less reliable, which can result in falsely high ankle pressures and a falsely elevated ABPI.

Exercise testing will assess the functional limitations of arterial stenoses and differentiate occlusive arterial disease from other causes of exercise-induced lower limb symptoms, e.g. neurogenic claudication secondary to spinal stenosis. A limited inflow of blood in a limb with occlusive arterial disease results in a fall in ankle SBP during exercise-induced peripheral vasodilatation. Patients can exercise for 5 min, ideally on a treadmill, but walking in the surgery or marking time on the spot are perfectly adequate. ABPI is measured before and after exercise. A pressure drop of ≥20% indicates significant arterial disease (Figure 1.4). If there is no drop in ankle SBP after a 5-min brisk walk, the patient does not have occlusive arterial disease proximal to the ankle in that limb.

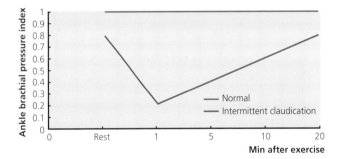

Figure 1.4 The fall in ABPI with exercise in a patient with intermittent claudication.

Duplex scanning

By combining the pulsed Doppler system with real-time B-mode ultrasound imaging of vessels, it is possible to examine (or 'sample') Doppler flow patterns in a precisely defined area within the vessel lumen. This combination of real-time B-mode sound imaging with pulsed Doppler ultrasound is called duplex scanning. The addition of colour frequency mapping makes the identification of arterial stenoses even easier and reduces scanning time (Figure 1.5).

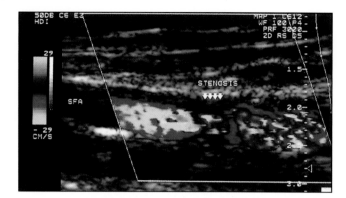

Figure 1.5 Colour duplex scanning of blood flow through a stenosis of the superficial femoral artery (SFA). The colour assignment (red or blue) depends on the direction of blood flow, and colour saturation reflects velocity of blood flow. Less saturation (mixed red and blue) indicates regions of higher blood flow, and deeper colours indicate slower flow; the absence of flow is coded as black.

Table 1.2 Uses of colour duplex scanning.

Arterial	Venous
Identify obstructive atherosclerotic disease: • Carotid • Peripheral arteries Surveillance of infrainguinal bypass grafts Surveillance of lower limb arteries after angioplasty	Diagnosis of deep vein thrombosis above the knee Assessing competence of valves in deep veins Superficial venous reflux: • Assessing patient with recurrent varicose veins • Identify and locate reflux at saphenopopliteal junction Pre-operative mapping of saphenous vein

In detecting femoral and popliteal disease, duplex ultrasonography has a sensitivity of 80% and a specificity of 90–100%, but ultrasound is less reliable for assessing the severity of stenoses in the tibial and peroneal arteries (Table 1.2). The National Institute of Clinical Excellence (NICE) advises the use of duplex scanning as first-line imaging to all people with suspected lower limb peripheral arterial disease for whom revascularisation is being considered (Box 1.1). Duplex scanning is especially useful for assessing the carotid arteries and for routine surveillance of infrainguinal bypass grafts where sites of stenosis can be identified before complete graft occlusion occurs and before there is a significant fall in ABPI. The normal velocity within a graft conduit ranges between

> **Box 1.1 NICE recommended imaging in patients with peripheral arterial disease in whom revascularisation is being considered**
>
> 1 Duplex U/S for first-line imaging
> 2 Contrast-enhanced MRA – if further imaging is required after initial U/S before considering revascularisation
> 3 CTA – if further imaging is required after initial U/S, if contrast-enhanced MRA is contraindicated or not tolerated, before considering revascularisation.

50 and 120 cm/s. As with native arteries, a 2-fold increase in peak systolic velocity indicates a stenosis of $\geq$50%. A peak velocity of <45 cm/s occurs in grafts at high risk of failure.

Computed tomography angiogram

CTA is a technique that allows rapid and continuous acquisition of data during the first pass of a bolus of i.v. contrast through the arterial tree. The data can be reconstructed at any slice level, reformatted into different planes and processed into high-quality two- or three-dimensional images of vessels. The introduction of multidetector computed tomography (MDCT) has had a dramatic effect on CT imaging, and, in particular, imaging of the cardiovascular system. The development of MDCT has led to a much higher speed of data acquisition (0.37-s rotation speed versus 1-s rotation speed for conventional CT), and, secondly, MDCT acquires volume data instead of individual slice data. Thus, MDCT (without increasing the radiation dose) has led to faster scanning, improved contrast resolution and better spatial resolution. The effect of movement artefacts is also minimised.

The time taken to complete the procedure is determined by practicalities such as transferring the patient and gaining venous access, but the scan acquisition time for the entire arterial system (aortic arch to pedal vessels) is <15 s for CTA compared with ~10–15 min for MRA (Table 1.3).

Magnetic resonance angiography

Certain MR scanning techniques allow the use of a pulse sequence that images moving blood, thus showing arteries or veins without the use of an injected contrast agent or exposure

Table 1.3 Advantages and limitations of CT and MR angiographies.

CTA	MRA (enhanced)
Rapid data acquisition; less prone to movement artefact	Slower acquisition; more prone to movement artefact
High resolution, providing anatomical images of the vessel lumen and wall	Lower resolution but dependent on technique and location
Loss of accuracy with circumferential calcification	May overestimate degree and length of stenosis due to signal dropout in areas of turbulence
Ease of access, especially in emergencies, and acutely ill patients can be supported during scan	Contraindicated by need for intensive patient support Contraindications include implants such as pacemakers, defibrillators, cochlear implants and spinal cord stimulators Small scanner tunnel not tolerated by some patients due to claustrophobia or body habitus
Less expensive	More expensive
Radiation exposure	No radiation
Iodinated contrast – risk of contrast nephropathy and allergy (effective hydration helps prevent nephropathy)	Gadolinium contrast used for MRA has been associated with nephrogenic systemic fibrosis (in patients with severe renal impairment)

to ionising radiation. Non-contrast MRA therefore has substantial safety advantages but is characterised by flow dependence. Contrast-enhanced MRA using an i.v. bolus of gadolinium contrast can cover a larger area, allows more rapid data acquisition and higher resolution and gives a more direct image of the vascular lumen. Therefore, contrast-enhanced MRA is more commonly used. A variety of imaging sequences are used depending on the vessels being studied and the field strength of the machine. Information is obtained from both the axial images and the vessel reconstructions (Figures 1.6 and 1.7).

Applications of CTA and MRA

CTA and MRA are both widely used to investigate large artery pathology (Figures 1.8 and 1.9). Each technique has different advantages and disadvantages (Table 1.3). CTA has the major advantage of speed, but local preferences and availability often determine which technique is used. Computed tomography pulmonary angiography (CTPA) for suspected pulmonary embolism (PE) is probably the most commonly used computerised angiographic investigation (Figure 1.10). CTPA is now recommended by NICE guidance as the first-line investigation for patients with a high risk of PE after clinical evaluation.

In the investigation of abdominal aortic aneurysm (AAA) and aortic dissection, CTA is the preferred investigation because it images the vessel wall and can provide information about mural thrombus, inflammatory changes and rupture. Software reconstructs hundreds of images and displays them in two- or three-dimensional planes (Figure 1.11). This becomes an important tool

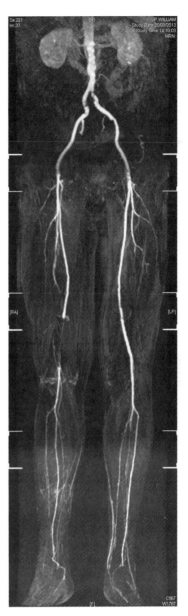

Figure 1.7 Contrast-enhanced MRA of the peripheral arteries showing bilateral common iliac stenosis and right superficial femoral artery occlusion.

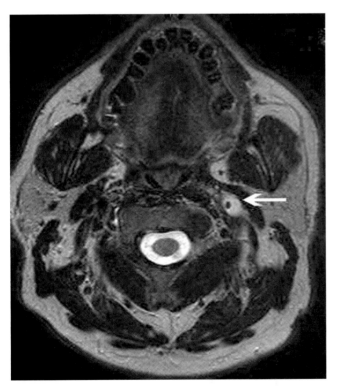

Figure 1.6 T2-weighted axial MR scan of the neck showing a left internal carotid artery dissection, with thrombus in the vessel wall producing a high signal (arrow).

for pre-operative planning and post-operative follow-up, especially in regard to use of endovascular stent grafts for AAA repair. CTA is more sensitive and specific than conventional angiography in detecting the presence of endoleaks.

Contrast-enhanced MRA is recommended in the investigation of suspected lower limb peripheral arterial disease for patients who need further imaging after initial duplex ultrasound before considering revascularisation. If MRA is contraindicated or not tolerated, patients should be offered CTA (Box 1.1).

MDCT angiography and MRA have equally high sensitivity and specificity for the detection of renal artery stenosis, but CTA is often preferred in order to avoid gadolinium administration, especially in patients with severe renal impairment (Figure 1.9). MDCT can also be used post stenting to assess for recurrent renal artery stenosis.

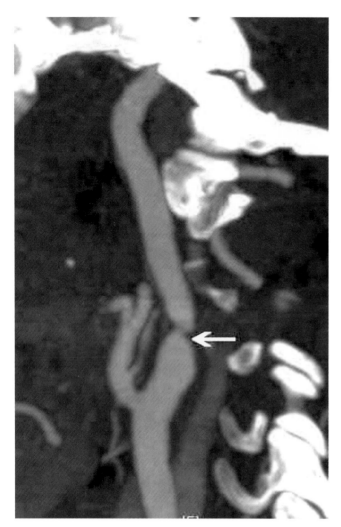

Figure 1.8 CT angiogram showing a tight stenosis of the right internal carotid artery (arrow).

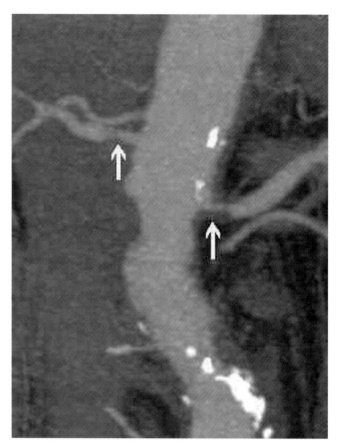

Figure 1.9 CT angiogram showing bilateral renal artery stenoses (arrows).

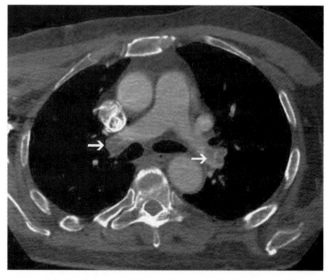

Figure 1.10 CT pulmonary angiogram showing a clot displacing contrast in both main pulmonary arteries (arrows).

Technical advances in both CT and MRI, with increased speed and resolution of imaging, coupled with data acquisition synchronised with respiratory and cardiac cycles, has led to their increased use in non-invasive cardiac imaging. Initial non-contrast CT is recommended to quantify calcification in the coronary arteries in patients with chest pain in whom clinical assessment and 12-lead ECG alone cannot diagnose angina and the likelihood of coronary artery disease (CAD) is low. The presence of calcium is a marker of atherosclerosis and there is a direct correlation between the extent of calcification of the coronary arteries and the risk of future cardiac events. If the 'calcium score' on CT is moderately elevated, contrast CTA of the coronary arteries is recommended and significant stenoses can be detected with a sensitivity of 95% or higher (Figure 1.12). MRI provides excellent anatomical and

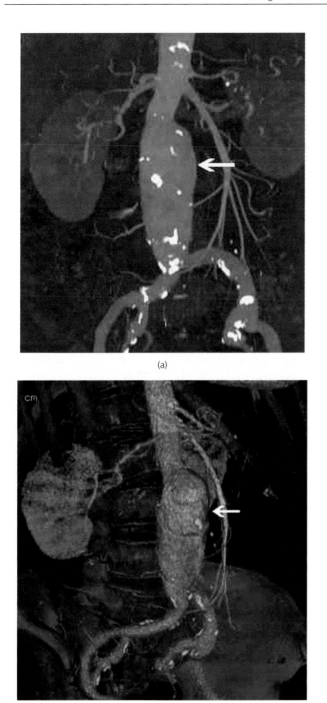

(a)

(b)

Figure 1.11 (a) CT angiogram showing an abdominal aortic aneurysm (arrow) and (b) the volume-rendered reconstruction of the CT angiogram in the same patient.

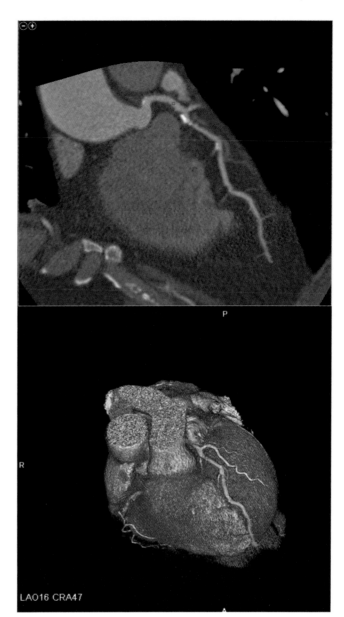

Figure 1.12 Calcified stenosis (arrow) of the proximal anterior descending branch of the left coronary artery.

functional cardiac detail. It can be used to characterise congenital heart disease, assess ventricular mass and function and differentiate forms of cardiomyopathy. Non-invasive functional cardiac MRI is recommended as an alternative to stress echocardiography or myocardial perfusion scintigraphy in the assessment of myocardial ischaemia using contrast-enhanced perfusion or stress-induced wall motion abnormality techniques.

Investigations in venous disease

Venous thrombosis

Colour duplex scanning is both sensitive and specific (90–100% in most series) for detecting proximal deep vein thrombosis (DVT).

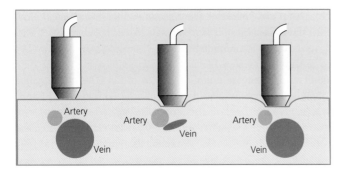

Figure 1.13 Ultrasound detection of a DVT. The probe is held lightly on the skin and advanced along the course of the vein (left). Pressure is applied every few centimetres by compressing the transducer head against the skin. The vein collapses during compression if no thrombus is present (middle) but not if a DVT is present (right).

Deep veins and arteries lie together in the leg, and the normal vein appears as an echo-free channel and is usually larger than the accompanying artery. Venous ultrasound has proved to be a very accurate method of identifying DVTs from the level of the common femoral vein at the groin crease to the popliteal vein, but the technique is much less reliable for diagnosing calf vein thrombosis (Figure 1.13). Approximately 40% of calf DVTs resolve spontaneously, 40% become organised and 20% propagate. Propagating DVT can be excluded by serial duplex scanning with an interval of 1 week.

Unenhanced or contrast magnetic resonance venography (MRV) is useful for examining the intracranial venous system, particularly in evaluating suspected dural venous sinus thrombosis. MRV and conventional enhanced (portal venous phase) CT can also be used to diagnose thrombus in intra-thoracic and abdominal veins.

Venous reflux

Colour duplex has revolutionised the investigation of the lower limb venous system because it allows instantaneous visualisation of blood flow and its direction. Thus, reflux at the saphenofemoral junction, saphenopopliteal junction and within the deep venous system, including the popliteal vein beneath the knee and the gastrocnemius veins, can be demonstrated non-invasively. Although a limited assessment of venous reflux can be undertaken using a pencil Doppler, compared with colour duplex the pencil Doppler misses ~12% of saphenofemoral and ~20% of saphenopopliteal junction reflux.

Further reading

Burrill J, Dabbagh Z, Gollub F, *et al.* Multidetector computed tomographic angiography of the cardiovascular system. *Postgrad Med J* 2007;**83**:698–704.

Chest Pain of recent onset; assessment and diagnosis of recent chest pain or discomfort of suspected cardiac origin NICE clinical guideline 95 March 2010.

Layden J, Michaels J, Bermingham S, and Higgins B, (on behalf of the clinical guideline development group). Diagnosis and management of lower limb peripheral arterial disease: summary of NICE guidance. *BMJ* 2012;**345**:42–43.

Orbell JH, Smith A, Burnand KG, *et al.* Imaging of deep vein thrombosis. *Br J Surg* 2008;**95**:37–136.

Ross R. Atherosclerosis – an inflammatory disease. *NEJM* 1999;**340**(2): 115–126.

Sheikh S, Gonzalez RG, Lev MH. Stroke CT angiography. In: Gonzalez RG, Hirsch JA, Koroshetz WJ *et al.*, eds. *Acute ischaemic stroke – imaging and intervention.* Springer, Berlin, 2006.

Stein PD, Hull RD. Multidetector computed tomography for the diagnosis of acute pulmonary embolism. *Curr Opin Pulm Med* 2007;**13**:384–388.

Venous thromboembolic diseases: the management of venous thromboembolic diseases and the role of thrombophilia testing NICE clinical guideline 144 June 2012.

CHAPTER 2

Cerebrovascular and Carotid Artery Disease

Timothy J. England[1], Nishath Altaf[2], and Shane MacSweeney[2]

[1] Division of Medical Sciences & GEM, School of Medicine, University of Nottingham, UK
[2] Department of Vascular Surgery, Nottingham University Hospitals NHS Trust, UK

OVERVIEW

- Stroke and transient ischaemic attack (TIA) are common medical emergencies
- Effective care requires rapid access to a specialist multidisciplinary team
- Thrombolysis for stroke under specialist supervision reduces disability
- Treatment and rehabilitation on a stroke unit reduces death, disability, complications and costs
- Modifiable risk factors are common and should be assessed systematically
- Carotid endarterectomy (CEA) is of proven major benefit in the management of selected patients with symptomatic carotid artery disease
- Delay to surgery after onset of symptoms greatly lessens the benefit conferred by CEA. If the delay exceeds 12 weeks, virtually no benefit accrues to the patient.

Introduction

Each year in the United Kingdom there are 150 000 new cases of stroke, more than one every 5 min. In 2010, it was the fourth largest cause of death (almost 50 000 cases), though mortality rates have halved in the past 20 years. TIA affects 35 per 100 000 population and has a high risk of subsequent stroke, particularly in the first month after the event. Therefore, both stroke and TIA should be referred immediately for specialist inpatient or outpatient assessment in order to institute measures that reduce the burden of subsequent disability and death. The cost to the UK economy, including direct healthcare, informal care costs and indirect costs is in the region of £9 billion.

Stroke is a clinical syndrome presenting with rapidly developing focal (or global) loss of cerebral function lasting for more than 24 h or leading to death, with no apparent cause other than that of vascular origin (World Health Organisation, 1978). A transient ischaemic attack (TIA) is traditionally defined as a sudden focal neurological deficit of the brain or eye, presumed to be of vascular origin and lasts less than 24 h. While this definition is valid and useful, it is based on the assumption that TIAs are associated with complete resolution of cerebral ischaemia with no permanent brain injury. Advances in acute stroke imaging have shown this to be false and a 'tissue-based' definition is often preferred. The typical duration of a TIA is less than 20 min.

Aetiology

TIAs and 85% of strokes are due to atherothrombotic occlusion of a cerebral artery or cardioembolism. Neurons are extremely oxygen dependent, and an irreversible process of cell death begins if perfusion is not quickly restored. Haemorrhage accounts for 15% of strokes, mainly from primary intracerebral haemorrhage due to small vessel lipohyalinosis. This causes tissue damage through compression and reactive vasospasm. However, one-third of patients may have an underlying tumour, aneurysm or arteriovenous malformation, so further investigations should be considered for those surviving without major disability. Stroke predominantly occurs in older people at an average age of 74, but 15% are under the age of 60 (Table 2.1). For younger patients, it is important to consider mechanisms other than atheroma for ischaemic stroke, such as carotid dissection, patent foramen ovale, thrombophilia and uncommon genetic disorders such as CADASIL (Cerebral Autosomal Dominant Arteriopathy with Subcortical Infarcts and Leucoencephalopathy) or Fabry's disease. However, no definitive cause is identified in one-third of patients despite investigations (Table 2.1).

Clinical assessment

The diagnosis of a stroke is initially based on a detailed history (taken from the patient or witness) and medical examination and confirmed with diagnostic radiological imaging. A typical history is one of a sudden loss of neurological function determined by the site of the brain that has been damaged by ischaemia or haemorrhage. Symptoms and signs (Table 2.2) are usually maximal at onset but occasionally they worsen gradually or in a stepwise manner. Alternative diagnoses (such as intracerebral malignancy) should be considered if ictus is not sudden. Unless there has been complete recovery at the time of medical review and the immediate risk of stroke is low, the patient should be admitted for neurological monitoring and urgent assessment. Stroke syndromes based on

ABC of Arterial and Venous Disease, Third Edition.
Edited by Tim England and Akhtar Nasim.
© 2015 John Wiley & Sons, Ltd. Published 2015 by John Wiley & Sons, Ltd.

Table 2.1 Important risk factors for ischaemic stroke and TIA.

	Clinical note	Assessment	First-line management
Atherothrombotic			
Hypertension	50% patients have systolic BP >160 mmHg at presentation	<130/80 is secondary prevention target	BP-lowering drugs and lifestyle advice
Diabetes mellitus	40% patients have moderate hyperglycaemia at presentation	Diagnose with fasting glucose, glucose tolerance test or HbA1c	Diet and glucose-lowering drugs
Hypercholesterolaemia	Check within 24 h of event	Treat if total cholesterol >4.0 mmol/l or LDL > 2 mmol/l	Statin
Smoking	Doubles the risk of stroke recurrence	Document pack years	Refer to smoking cessation service
Carotid artery stenosis	Adhere to local protocol for carotid ultrasound	Considering treating symptomatic stenosis of 50–99%	Carotid endarterectomy
Carotid dissection	Neck pain and Horner's syndrome	CT or MR angiography of neck vessels	Anticoagulation or antiplatelet drugs for 3–6 months
Thrombophilia	Reserve for younger patients without vascular risk factors	Thrombophilia screen	Consider anticoagulation
Cardioembolic			
Atrial fibrillation	Consider 24-h ECG	ECG	Long-term anticoagulation
Recent myocardial infarct (MI)	Highest risk is anterior MI <4 weeks	ECG Transthoracic echocardiogram	Anticoagulation for 3–6 months
Left ventricular aneurysm	ECG with ST elevation	Transthoracic echocardiogram	Long-term anticoagulation
Patent foramen ovale	Younger patients without vascular risk factors	Transoesophageal echocardiogram	Consider closure or anticoagulation if aneurismal atrial septal defect and/or previous events

Table 2.2 Typical clinical features of a stroke or TIA.

Symptom	Descriptive term
Motor symptoms	
Weakness of one side of the body	Hemiparesis
Difficulty swallowing	Dysphagia
Imbalance	Ataxia
Inability to perform certain actions not due to weakness	Dyspraxia
Sensory symptoms	
Altered feeling on one side of the body	Hemisensory disturbance
Neglect of one side	Tactile or visual inattention
Loss of vision in one eye	Monocular blindness or amaurosis fugax
Loss of vision in a visual field	Hemianopia or quadrantanopia
Double vision	Diplopia
A spinning sensation	Vertigo
Speech or language disturbance	
Difficulty understanding or expressing spoken language	Receptive or expressive dysphasia
Difficulty writing	Dysgraphia
Difficulty calculating	Dyscalculia
Slurred speech	Dysarthria

clinical features, established by the Oxfordshire Community Stroke Project (OCSP), allow the clinician to estimate information on the anatomical and vascular location of the stroke, its aetiology and prognosis (Box 2.1). Many conditions can present in a similar way to stroke (Box 2.2). Particular care should be taken when there is a global disturbance of consciousness as this hinders identification of precise neurological deficits and increases the probability of an alternative mechanism for any focal signs.

> **Box 2.1 The Oxford Clinical Stroke Project (OCSP) classification of stroke**
>
> **1 Total anterior circulation syndrome (TACS)**
> a. Hemiparesis involving at least two of face, arm and leg, with or without hemisensory loss
> b. homonymous hemianopia and
> c. cortical (or 'higher cerebral') dysfunction, usually a dysphasia if involving the dominant hemisphere or inattention/neglect if involving the non-dominant hemisphere.
>
> These are usually large infarcts involving the middle cerebral or anterior cerebral artery or due to large lobar haematoma. Prognosis is poor with 60% dead and 35% dependent at 1 year post stroke.
>
> **2 Partial anterior circulation syndrome (PACS)**
> a. A combination of two of the three features of a TACS
> b. isolated high cerebral dysfunction or
> c. sensory motor deficit isolated to one of the face, arm or leg.
>
> PACS are usually secondary to occlusion of one of the branches of the middle cerebral or anterior cerebral arteries or due to lobar haemorrhage, with 15% dead and 30% dependent at 1 year.
>
> **3 Lacunar syndrome (LACS)**
> There are four main LACSs:
> a. Pure motor hemiparesis (up to 50% of lacunar cases) causes unilateral weakness of two of three of face, arm or leg. The lesion often occurs in the internal capsule or pons.
> b. Pure hemisensory *loss* (less common). The lesion is usually in the thalamus.

   c. Hemisensorimotor loss (35% of lacunar cases). The lesion may be in the thalamus, internal capsule, corona radiata or pons.
   d. Ataxic hemiparesis (10% of lacuna cases) is a combination weakness and ataxia in the arm and/or leg. The responsible lesion is usually in the pons, internal capsule or cerebral peduncle.

Prognosis is fair with 10% dead and 30% dependent at 1 year.

4 Posterior circulation syndrome (POCS)

Strokes involving the posterior circulation include those affecting the brainstem, cerebellum, thalamus or occipital lobe and can cause multiple signs and syndromes (e.g. isolated hemianopia and cranial nerve palsies, lateral medullary syndrome, and 'locked-in' syndrome). Sixty percent are independent at 1 year.

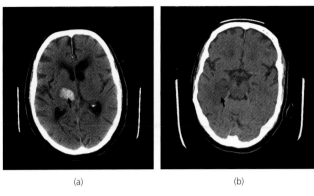

(a)   (b)

Figure 2.1 The appearance of acute haemorrhage and ischaemic stroke on CT imaging. (a) Hyperdense area representing blood. (b) Hypodense area representing infarction.

Box 2.2 **Common stroke mimics**

- Seizures
- Syncope
- Sepsis
- Somatisation
- Space-occupying lesion
- Sugar (hypoglycaemia and hyperglycaemia)
- Subdural (including unwitnessed head trauma)
- Single nerve injury (including Bell's palsy)
- Severe migraine
- Sclerosis (demyelination).

Diagnostic imaging

A computerised tomography (CT) or magnetic resonance (MR) brain scan should be performed as soon as possible and immediately (next available slot) in suspected stroke if any of the following apply:

- Indications for thrombolysis or early anticoagulation
- A depressed level of consciousness (Glasgow coma score <13)
- On anticoagulation treatment or a known bleeding tendency
- Unexplained progressive or fluctuating symptoms
- Severe headache at onset
- Papilloedema, fever or neck stiffness.

Both CT and MR scans are equally effective at detecting acute haemorrhage but a CT scan is usually the initial investigation of choice because it is more widely available, less expensive and safer to use in acutely ill stroke patients (Figure 2.1). When there is uncertainty about diagnosis, magnetic resonance imaging (MRI) with diffusion-weighted imaging (DWI) is very useful as it is highly specific for cerebral ischaemia within the previous 7–10 days (Figure 2.2). Advanced CT or MRI with angiography and perfusion imaging is increasingly being used to identify patients most suitable for thrombolytic therapy.

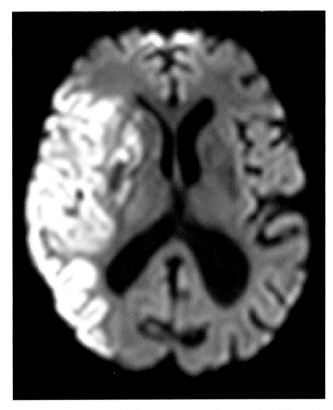

Figure 2.2 Diffusion-weighted MRI appearance of a recent large ischaemic stroke in the right middle cerebral artery.

Emergency management

Stroke is a medical emergency and should be treated with the same urgency as acute myocardial infarction. Acute stroke care begins in the community with recognition of a 'brain attack'; educating paramedics can increase their diagnostic accuracy and lead to an increase in the rates of thrombolysis. A useful aid to enhance recognition within the community, particularly for paramedics, is the FAST (face arm speech time) test that shows good agreement

SPINAL BOARD
R.E.D.
VACUUM MAT

CERVICAL COLLAR
ORTHO. STRETCHER
OTHER

11.STROKE (FACE ARM SPEECH TEST)

SPEECH IMPAIRMENT	YES	NO
FACIAL PALSY	YES	NO
AFFECTED SIDE	L	R
ARM WEAKNESS?	YES	NO
AFFECTED SIDE	L	R

12.CANNULATION
SIZE   14g   16g   18g

Figure 2.3 The FAST on an ambulance report form.

Assessment   Date ☐☐☐☐☐☐   Time ☐☐☐☐

Symptom onset Date ☐☐☐☐☐☐   Time ☐☐☐☐

GCS E=☐ M=☐ V=☐   BP ☐☐   *BM ☐

*IF BM<3.5mmol/L treat urgently and reassess once blood glucose normal

Has there been loss of consciousness or syncope?   Y(−1)☐ N(0)☐

Has there been seizure activity?   Y(−1)☐ N(0)☐

Is there a <u>NEW ACUTE</u> onset (or on awakening from sleep)

I.   Asymmetric facial weakness   Y(+1)☐ N(0)☐

II. Asymmetric arm weakness   Y(+1)☐ N(0)☐

III. Asymmetric leg weakness   Y(+1)☐ N(0)☐

IV. Speech disturbance   Y(+1)☐ N(0)☐

V.   Visual field defect   Y(+1)☐ N(0)☐

*Total Score _____ (−2 to +5)

Provision diagnosis

☐ Stoke ☐ Non-stroke (specify) _____

*Stroke is unlikely but not completely excluded if total scores are ≤ 0.

Figure 2.4 The ROSIER score.

with physician assessment (Figure 2.3). A similar tool is available for emergency department staff (ROSIER score; Figure 2.4).

Occlusion of a major cerebral artery leads to a severe reduction in cerebral blood flow (CBF). Cell death then occurs at a rate of ~1.9 million neurons per minute. CBF reduction is greatest at the core of the ischaemic area where there is metabolic failure and cell death. Surrounding the core is an area of tissue at risk of death (the ischaemic penumbra; Figure 2.5), but the reduction in CBF is less severe due to collateral blood supply. The cells become dysfunctional when CBF falls below 0.16–0.17 mls/g/min. Hence, many therapeutic and experimental interventions attempt to re-establish CBF sufficiently to prevent cell death in the penumbra.

Administration of intravenous recombinant tissue plasminogen activator (rt-PA, alteplase) within 4.5 h of onset reduces disability by restoring perfusion to acutely ischaemic areas; an additional 90 patients will achieve independence for every 1000 treated. The reduction in infarct size is offset by an increased risk of intracranial haemorrhage, of which approximately 5% are symptomatic (2–3% fatal). Earlier administration confers greater benefit and a lower risk of bleeding. Currently, there is no clear evidence to suggest that intra-arterial thrombolysis or mechanical thrombectomy are superior to intravenous therapy though they are performed in selected cases. Administration of aspirin is usually delayed for 24 h post thrombolysis.

Patients with primary intracerebral haemorrhage (PICH) do not routinely benefit from surgical intervention, although individual cases should be discussed with the local neurosurgical service (Table 2.3). Recent evidence suggests that lowering blood pressure acutely in patients with PICH is safe and probably improves long-term outcome.

Stroke unit care

All stroke patients should be admitted to an acute stroke unit as soon as possible. Organised stroke unit care, compared to general wards, reduces the odds of death or dependency (by 21%), the need for institutionalised care and are more cost effective. They also provide palliative care for a small number of patients because of stroke severity and pre-existing co-morbidities.

The stroke unit facilitates recovery by using organised multidisciplinary care, involving doctors, nurses, physiotherapists, occupational therapists, speech and language therapists, dieticians, psychologists, social workers and pharmacists. The length of stay

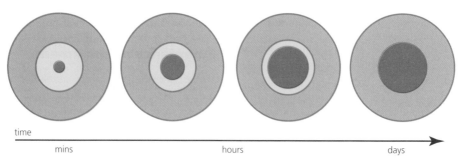

time

mins   hours   days

Figure 2.5 Schematic of the ischaemic penumbra. An area of ischaemic but potentially viable tissue surrounds an infarct core. Over time, the core grows at the cost of the penumbra. The blue area represents the brain; yellow, the penumbra; red, the infarct core.

Table 2.3 Indications for neuroscience consultation.

Scenario	Possible intervention
Suspected basilar artery thrombosis <24 h	Intra-arterial thrombolysis
Superficial primary intracerebral haemorrhage with further neurological deterioration	Surgical evacuation if early and patient is conscious Hydrocephalus treatment
Haemorrhage with suspected underlying aneurysm	Angiography and clipping or radiological coiling
Conscious level deterioration following posterior fossa haematoma	Surgical evacuation and hydrocephalus treatment
Conscious level deterioration following large MCA infarct (malignant MCA infarction due to oedema)	Decompressive craniectomy if early and no significant co-morbidities

MCA, middle cerebral artery.

Table 2.4 Risk of stroke after TIA.

ABCD^2 score		Total score	Stroke risk (%)		
Feature	Score		2 day	7 day	90 day
Age ≥60	1	0–3 (low risk)	1.0	1.2	3.1
Blood pressure ≥140/90	1	4–5 (moderate risk)	4.1	5.9	9.8
Clinical features		6–7 (high risk)	8.1	11.7	17.8
Unilateral weakness	2				
Speech disturbance	1				
Duration					
≥1 h	2				
10–59 min	1				
Diabetes	1				

Adapted from Johnston *et al.* (2007). Reproduced by permission of Elsevier.

should be tailored to individual needs, using goal-based therapy, allowing progress to be measured. Complications such as deep vein thrombosis and pulmonary embolus (preventable by intermittent pneumatic compression to the legs), infections, recurrent stroke, seizures, pressure ulcers, incontinence, pain, spasticity and post-stroke depression can often inhibit targeted goals. The overall aim is to minimise handicap and return the patient to an optimal functional state. Many patients can be discharged home earlier if there is a community-based specialist team to continue with personal care assistance and rehabilitation.

Feeding

Swallowing is initially impaired following stroke in ~50% of patients, although many can manage safe oral intake of a modified diet under nursing supervision with speech therapy guidance. Temporary nasogastric feeding should be started within 24–48 h of stroke in conscious patients who cannot demonstrate safe swallowing. Good oral care is paramount. There is no significant survival advantage from insertion of a percutaneous endoscopic gastrostomy (PEG) tube earlier than 1 month, as swallowing will often improve quickly for many patients, while those with severe swallowing problems have a high early mortality related to the underlying stroke severity.

Secondary prevention

All patients require a review of cardiovascular risk factors, particularly blood pressure, glucose and cholesterol levels. In the absence of a cardioembolic source, ischaemic stroke and TIA should be treated with antiplatelets; clopidogrel monotherapy is the current preferred option that has equal efficacy and a slightly lower bleeding risk than combined aspirin and dipyridamole. Patients with atrial fibrillation or another cardioembolic cause should be anticoagulated soon after the event unless major contraindications are present.

The stroke risk following TIA can be effectively estimated by use of the ABCD^2 score (Table 2.4). Patients scoring ≥4 have a stroke risk of >4% in the next 48 h and so require an urgent specialist review. Screening for carotid stenosis by ultrasound should be

offered to high-risk patients with carotid territory TIA within 24 h and those who have recovered independence in personal care following anterior circulation ischaemic stroke.

Carotid endarterectomy

Extracranial carotid stenosis accounts for 20–30% of all strokes and asymptomatic carotid stenosis is found in about 7% of women and 12% of men older than 70 years. The overriding mechanism of stroke in patients with carotid disease remains thromboembolism of atherothrombotic debris from a stenotic carotid plaque (Figures 2.6 and 2.7). Carotid endarterectomy (CEA) is a well-established procedure that removes the source of embolisation, namely, the plaque from the carotid artery. An alternative procedure involves placing a stent across the carotid plaque (CAS, carotid artery stenting). Both, however, have their own risk of complications that need to be balanced against the risk of a stroke with best medical therapy.

Evidence for treating symptomatic patients with CEA

CEA is one of the most scientifically scrutinised surgical procedures of all time. Table 2.5 summarises the principle outcomes from the Carotid Endarterectomy Trialists Collaboration (CETC) who combined data from more than 6000 patients randomised into the three main symptomatic trials. Table 2.5 also includes parallel data from the two multicentre randomised trials [ACAS (asymptomatic carotid artery stenosis) and ACST (asymptomatic carotid surgery trial)] comparing outcomes in asymptomatic patients.

In symptomatic patients, the CETC observed that CEA conferred a modest but significant benefit in patients with 50–69% stenosis. This equates to a relative risk reduction (RRR) of 28%, a number needed to treat (NNT) of 13 and 78 strokes prevented at 5 years by performing 1000 CEAs. The greatest benefit, however, was observed in patients with 70–99% stenosis (RRR = 48%, NNT = 6 and 156 strokes will be prevented at 5 years by performing 1000 CEAs).

One of the most important subgroup analyses to come from the CETC (Table 2.6) was recognition that while the trials recruited patients who had been symptomatic within the preceding 6 months,

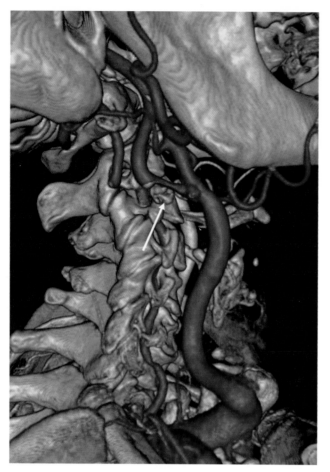

Figure 2.6 Three-dimensional CT angiogram showing a severe stenosis of the internal carotid artery (arrowed) just distal to the bifurcation.

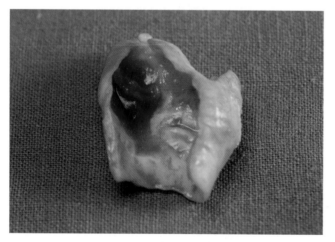

Figure 2.7 Carotid endarterectomy specimen showing the excised plaque with overlying thrombus. Embolisation of this thrombotic material is responsible for 50% of ischaemic carotid territory TIAs and strokes.

Table 2.5 Carotid Endarterectomy Trialists Collaboration: 5-year risk of stroke (including 30-day stroke/death) from (i) the CETC analysis of the symptomatic randomised trials and (ii) the ACAS and ACST asymptomatic randomised trials.

Trial	Stenosis (%)	30-day CEA risk (%)	5-year risk surgery (%)	Medical (%)	RRR (%)	NNT	Strokes prevented per 1000 CEAs
CETC	<30		18.4	15.7	n/b	n/b	None at 5 years
CETC	30–49	6.7	22.8	25.4	10	38	26 at 5 years
CETC	50–69	8.4	20.0	27.8	28	13	78 at 5 years
CETC	70–99	6.2	17.1	32.7	48	6	156 at 5 years
CETC	String sign	5.4	22.4	22.3	n/b	n/b	None at 5 years
ACST	60–99	2.8	6.4	11.8	46	19	53 at 5 years
ACAS	60–99	2.3	5.1	11.0	54	17	59 at 5 years

30-day CEA risk, 30-day risk of death/stroke after CEA; n/b, no benefit conferred by CEA; RRR, relative risk reduction; NNT, number needed to treat to prevent one stroke; strokes prevented per 1000 CEAs, number of strokes prevented at 5 years by performing 1000 CEAs.

Table 2.6 CETC: effect of delay from randomisation to surgery on actual benefit conferred by CEA.

	<2 weeks	2–4 weeks	4–12 weeks	>12 weeks
ARR at 5 years	18.5%	9.8%	5.5%	0.8%
NNT at 5 years	5	10	18	125

ARR at 5 years, absolute risk reduction in stroke conferred by CEA at 5 years compared with best medical therapy; NNT, number of CEAs to be performed to prevent one stroke at 5 years.

Table 2.7 Which symptomatic patients gain most benefit from carotid endarterectomy?

Clinical features	Imaging features
Males vs females	Ulcerated/irregular stenoses
Hemispheric vs retinal symptoms	Increasing stenosis (but not near occlusion)
Recurrent symptoms for >6 months	Contralateral occlusion
Very recent symptoms (2 weeks)	Tandem intracranial disease
Increasing medical co-morbidity	
Increasing age	
Very rapid surgery	

the maximum benefit was observed in patients who had undergone surgery within 2 weeks of randomisation. The absolute risk reduction (ARR) in stroke at 5 years was 18.5% in patients undergoing surgery within 2 weeks (NNT = 5), falling to just 0.8% if the surgery was deferred for >12 weeks (NNT = 125). Moreover, females gained less benefit (than males) from CEA, especially if the surgery was deferred for >4 weeks. Table 2.7 summarises other secondary analyses from the international randomised trials that identified patients who gained most benefit from intervention. The ECST (European carotid surgery trial) risk model utilises such parameters to calculate estimated stroke rates in different groups of patients presenting with carotid disease (www.stroke.ox.ac.uk).

In summary:

• The quicker the operation is performed, the greater the long-term benefit. Excessive delays will expose some patients to all of the procedural risks with little prospect of benefit.

- Age is no bar to surgery. In the international trials, patients aged >75 years gained more benefit than any other age group.
- Patients exhibiting near occlusion (string sign) do not seem to benefit from CEA.
- Finally, the higher the risk of intervention, the less the long-term benefit. All surgical units must therefore maintain a rigorous audit of outcomes. The 30-day death/stroke rates should be <5% in standard risk symptomatic patients and <3% in asymptomatic individuals.

Evidence for treating asymptomatic patients with CEA

In asymptomatic patients, both ACAS and ACST trials showed that immediate CEA (as opposed to deferred CEA) was associated with a small but significant reduction in the risk of late stroke, from ~12% at 5 years to ~6% (Table 2.5). On average, 18 patients need to undergo surgery to prevent one stroke at 5 years and, provided the 30-day risk remains <2.5%, approximately 56 strokes will be prevented at 5 years by performing 1000 operations. CEA for asymptomatic patients does not appear to benefit patients >75 years and women do not benefit as much as men.

However, results from cohort studies showed that the incidence rate of stroke was low, particularly in studies carried out in the last decade, with stroke rates being 1.13% per year due to improving medical management. There is certainly significant controversy in the treatment of this subgroup of patients as the benefit from surgery is much less than that for symptomatic patients. Currently, UK guidelines suggest that surgery in asymptomatic patients should only be offered as part of a trial.

Treatment of carotid disease with carotid artery stenting

CAS (Figure 2.8) has emerged as a non-invasive alternative to CEA, and quoted advantages include no neck incision, no cranial nerve injuries, shorter hospital stay and improved cost-effectiveness. It is inevitable that CAS and CEA will have a complementary role but, to date, a number of randomised trials have failed to establish consensus.

The 2013 Cochrane review of 16 trials involving >7500 patients randomised to CEA or CAS showed that in symptomatic patients, CAS was associated with a higher risk of 30-day stroke or death and had a higher rate of restenosis. This was particularly true in patients older than 70 years of age. However, CAS was associated with lower risks of myocardial infarction, cranial nerve palsy and haematomas. The long-term rates of strokes were similar in both groups. The authors of the Cochrane review do recommend that CEA should be offered to symptomatic patients over 70 years of age and that CAS may be offered to younger patients at centres achieving peri-operative stroke rates that are comparable to those with CEA.

In asymptomatic patients, there were no significant differences in the 30-day stroke rates between the two groups. The ACST-2 trial and the ECST-2 trial are currently investigating outcomes

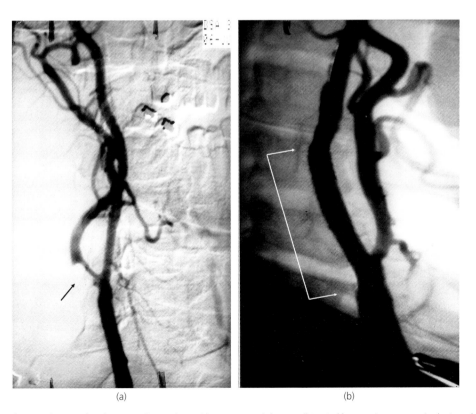

(a)   (b)

Figure 2.8 (a) Pre-angioplasty angiogram showing severe internal carotid artery stenosis (arrowed) treated by percutaneous angioplasty and stenting (b, arrowed).

of asymptomatic patients undergoing intervention and best medical therapy.

Conclusion

Stroke and TIA are medical emergencies requiring rapid assessment by a multiprofessional team. The evidence for strategies to prevent and reduce the consequences of cerebrovascular disease continues to grow, but patients and society will only benefit if specialist services are implemented and accessed in a timely manner.

Clinical scenario: a patient presenting with a transient ischaemic attack

Presentation: A 76-year-old man presented to his GP with sudden loss of vision affecting his left eye that had occurred on two occasions 2 days previously. He had also noticed several episodes of loss of sensation and power in the right hand and arm, most recently earlier that day he dropped his cup of tea and was unable to pick it up again. This lasted about 20 min. He was a smoker with a history of ischaemic heart disease and COPD (chronic obstructive pulmonary disease). He was already taking antiplatelets and a statin.

Examination findings: He was alert and orientated with no neurological abnormality. He was in sinus rhythm, pulse 82, BP 140/90.

Diagnosis: TIA.

Investigations: He was referred to the TIA clinic on the same day and underwent an MRI brain scan, ECG, FBC and ESR glucose U and E, and a carotid duplex scan.

Results: ECG and blood tests were normal, MRI showed no focal abnormality, with carotid duplex 80% stenosis in left internal carotid origin.

Management: Referred to vascular surgeons and underwent uneventful left carotid endarterectomy on the following day.

Outcome: Discharged home on the morning after surgery.

Further reading

Johnston SC, Rothwell PM, Nguyen-Huynh MN *et al.* Validation and refinement of scores to predict very early stroke risk after transient ischaemic attack. *Lancet* 2007;**369**:283–292.

Nor AM, Davis J, Sen B *et al.* The recognition of stroke in the emergency room (ROSIER) scale: development and validation of a stroke recognition instrument. *Lancet Neurol* 2005;**4**:727–734.

Royal College of Physicians. *National clinical guideline for stroke*, 4th edn. Prepared by the Intercollegiate Stroke Working Party. RCP, London, 2012.

Stroke Unit Trialists' Collaboration. Organised inpatient (stroke unit) care for stroke. Cochrane Database of Systematic Reviews 2013, Issue 9. Art. No.: CD000197. DOI: 10.1002/14651858.CD000197.pub3.

Wardlaw JM, Murray V, Berge E *et al.* Recombinant tissue plasminogen activator for acute ischaemic stroke: an updated systematic review and meta-analysis. *Lancet* 2012;**379**:2364–2372.

Rerkasem K and Rothwell PM. Carotid endarterectomy for symptomatic carotid stenosis. Cochrane Database of Systematic Reviews 2011, Issue 4. Art. No.: CD001081. DOI: 10.1002/14651858.CD001081.pub2.

CHAPTER 3

Coronary Artery Disease and Acute Coronary Syndrome

Asif Adnan[1] and David Adlam[2]

[1] Royal Derby Hospital, UK
[2] Department of cardiovascular Sciences, University of Leicester, UK

OVERVIEW

- Ischaemic heart disease is the single most common cause of death in the developed world
- Preventive measures and risk factor modification are a key part of current clinical management
- Treatment of symptomatic patients includes both pharmacological and invasive approaches
- Immediate reperfusion (usually by primary angioplasty) in STEMI (ST-elevation myocardial infarction) is the prime aim of early treatment and heavily relies on accurate early diagnosis and prompt clinical intervention
- This chapter is aimed at providing an insight to the non-specialist about various cardiac investigations and management strategies in everyday practice.

Epidemiology

The global burden of coronary disease is still rising. In the United Kingdom, ischaemic heart disease remains the most common cause of mortality among men and women, accounting for approximately 64 000 deaths in the year 2012. This translates to around 1 in 6 deaths in men and 1 in 10 deaths in women. However, a better understanding and control of risk factors (primary prevention) along with advancement in treatment strategies has nearly halved death rates over the past 10 years (Office of National Statistics, United Kingdom).

Pathophysiology

Clinically, coronary artery disease presents either acutely with myocardial infarction (MI) or chronically with stable angina. Stable angina occurs when progressive coronary stenosis leads to an insufficiency of myocardial blood supply, particularly at times of increased myocardial metabolic demand, such as on exercise. This leads to myocardial ischaemia and symptomatic angina (Figure 3.1a). MI results from acute occlusive thrombus formation at the site of an atherosclerotic plaque leading to myocardial

ischaemia or infarction. This frequently results from a disruption at sites where the fibrous cap overlying atherosclerotic plaque is thinned. This exposes prothrombotic elements of the necrotic core to the flowing coronary blood triggering platelet activation aggregation and subsequent thrombus formation (Figure 3.1b). Over time, areas of atherosclerosis become increasingly calcified.

Risk factors

The non-modifiable risk factors for coronary artery disease are advanced age, male sex and family history. The modifiable risks are tobacco smoking, dyslipidaemia, hypertension, diabetes mellitus, truncal obesity, dietary habits, alcohol consumption and physical activity. Together these account for >90% of the risk of an MI. Understanding of the role of genetic factors in determining risk may become an important element of patient risk profiling. The risk of a cardiovascular event can be estimated using calculations derived from previous population studies (example shown in Figure 3.2)

Management of risk factors

For both primary and secondary prevention of coronary disease, patients should be given advice and support for smoking cessation, better dietary habits and an active life style. Hypertension, hyperlipidaemia and diabetes should be treated with the aim of achieving therapeutic targets (Table 3.1).

Chronic stable angina

History

The classical description of 'Angina Pectoris' is of a constrictive retrosternal pain with or without radiation to the arm or jaw that comes on exertion and relieves with rest or sublingual nitrate. However, chest pain is a common presenting symptom (2.5–3% of all emergency room attendance) and there is considerable variation in patients' description of angina. A low index of suspicion is therefore required. Some patients present without chest pain describing only exertional breathlessness, a condition termed 'angina equivalent'. The key element of the history is usually a limitation of exercise capacity due to chest discomfort and/or breathlessness (although even this may be difficult to gauge in

ABC of Arterial and Venous Disease, Third Edition.
Edited by Tim England and Akhtar Nasim.
© 2015 John Wiley & Sons, Ltd. Published 2015 by John Wiley & Sons, Ltd.

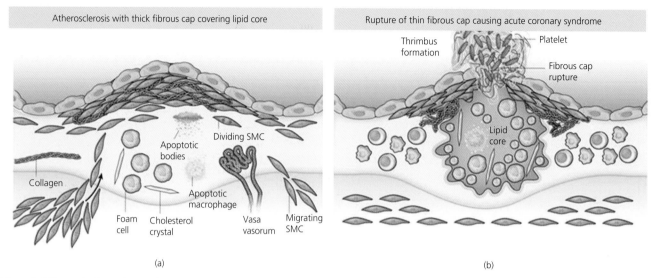

Atherosclerosis with thick fibrous cap covering lipid core

Rupture of thin fibrous cap causing acute coronary syndrome

(a)

(b)

Figure 3.1 Types of atherosclerotic plaque. (a) Atherosclerotic plaques with thicker fibrous caps are less likely to rupture but may lead to coronary stenosis restricting coronary blood flow and causing stable angina when myocardial oxygen demand is high. (b) Atherosclerotic plaques with a large necrotic core and thin fibrous cap are vulnerable to rupture triggering platelet activation and thrombus formation leading to an acute coronary syndrome. Source: Adapted from Libby *et al.* (2011). Reproduced by permission of Nature Publishing Group.

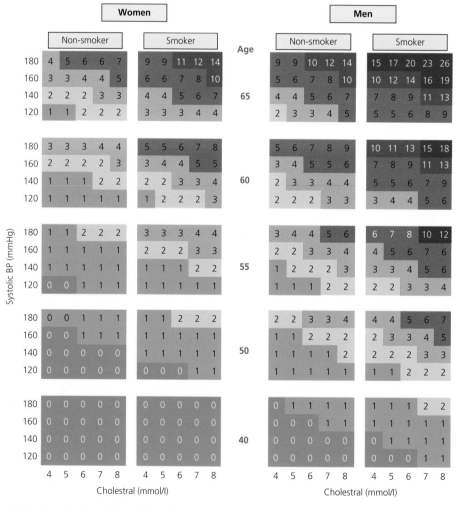

Figure 3.2 Example of a risk calculator for determining patient risk on the basis of common risk factors. A cell is identified for a given patient based on age, sex, systolic BP, cholesterol level and smoking status. This gives the percentage risk over 10 years. Risk is higher than estimated in patients with obesity, sedentary life style, family history of premature CVD, ethnic minority with poorer socioeconomic background, chronic kidney disease, low HDL (high-density lipoprotein) and high triglycerides. Source: Adapted from Conroy *et al.* (2003). Reproduced by permission of Oxford University Press.

Table 3.1 Therapeutic targets for common risk factors for subjects at high risk of coronary artery disease.

Risk factor	Ideal target
Hypertension	
Diabetic	130/80 mmHg
Non-diabetic	140/85 mmHg
Diabetes	HBA1c < 6.5%
Hyperlipidaemia	
Total cholesterol	<4 mmol/L or >25% reduction
LDL	<2 mmol/L or >30% reduction

This includes patients with established atherosclerotic disease, asymptomatic individuals with estimated CVD (cardiovascular disease) risk of ≥ 20% over 10 years and any patient with diabetes.

patients with poor mobility). The clinical pretest probability can be further enhanced by a detailed assessment of risk factors. This will then guide decision making on treatment including therapeutic risk factor modification and further investigations with a view to potential coronary revascularisation.

Physical examination

A patient with angina often will have no abnormality on physical examination. But features of risk factors such as nicotine staining, xanthelasma, hypertension and signs of end organ damage from

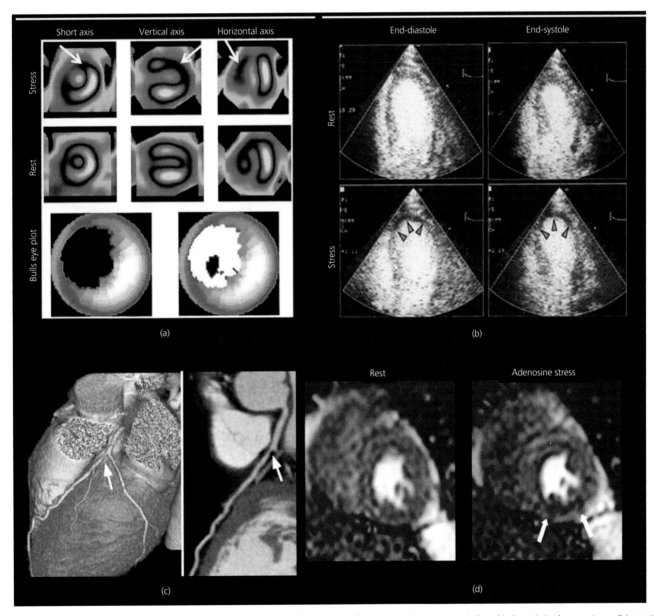

Figure 3.3 Different diagnostic modalities for coronary artery disease. (a) Nuclear perfusion scan showing stress-induced ischaemia in the anterior wall (arrow). Source: Adapted from Sabharwal and Lahiri (2003). Reproduced by permission of BMJ Publishing Group Ltd. (b) Dipyridamole stress echocardiography showing antero-apical ischaemia (arrow). Source: Adapted from Armstrong and Zoghbi (2005). Reproduced by permission of Elsevier. (c) Multiplane CT coronary angiography showing proximal LAD stenosis (arrow). (d) Adenosine stress MRI showing inferior wall ischaemia (arrow). Source: Adapted from Jhanke *et al.* (2006). Reproduced by permission of Wolters Kluwer Health.

diabetes may be present. Cardiovascular examination might reveal signs of heart failure, valvular disease or peripheral vascular disease.

Investigation

Simple investigations such as blood pressure, blood sugar and cholesterol and urine dip stick are invaluable in detecting otherwise unknown risk factors.

A resting 12-lead electrocardiograph (ECG) should be performed. This may show markers of hypertension (e.g. signs of left ventricular hypertrophy), evidence of old MI (e.g. pathological Q waves). A normal ECG does not exclude clinically important coronary artery disease.

A chest radiograph may show cardiomegaly, pulmonary congestion and will assess the non-cardiac structures for other potential explanation of the symptoms.

The next stage of investigation is aimed at confirming diagnosis and deciding whether or not to proceed to coronary angiography. The choice of investigation depends on the clinical pretest probability. The mainstay of investigation until recently was the exercise ECG. Although this test is still widely used, it is limited by relatively low specificity and sensitivity in the setting of diagnosing angina. The gold standard anatomical test for coronary artery disease is angiography; this is an invasive procedure and is associated with a small procedural risk. In patients with a very high pretest probability, it remains appropriate to proceed directly to angiography. However, in those with intermediate pretest probabilities, a number of non-invasive tests have been developed to determine which patients should proceed to angiography. These can be divided into anatomical tests such as computed tomography (CT) coronary calcium scoring and CT angiography that is most effective at discriminating those at the lower end of pretest risk and functional tests such as stress echocardiography, stress magnetic resonance imaging (MRI) and myocardial perfusion scintography that are most effective in those with intermediate pretest risk (Figure 3.3). The relative role of each imaging modality in the diagnosis of stable coronary disease remains subject to ongoing research and the current UK NICE (National Institute for Health and Clinical

Table 3.2 Investigating stable chest pain.

Clinical assessment	First-line diagnostic test
Features of typical angina and estimated likelihood of CAD >90%*	None required, manage as angina
Stable angina cannot be excluded on clinical assessment alone and	
Estimated likelihood of CAD is 61–90%*	Invasive coronary angiography
Estimated likelihood of CAD is 30–60%*	Non-invasive functional imaging (e.g. MPS, cardiac stress MRI and stress echo)
Estimated likelihood of CAD is 10–29%*	CT calcium scoring

*See NICE clinical guideline 95 (CG95 March 2010); MPS, myocardial perfusion scintigraphy.

Effectiveness) recommended strategy is summarised in Table 3.2. A summary of the overall approach is presented in Box 3.1.

> Box 3.1 **Assessing a patient with suspected coronary artery disease**
>
> Clinical assessment of patients with suspected coronary artery disease:
>
> - A careful history with emphasis on risk factors and characteristics of symptoms
> - A focussed clinical examination
> - Simple and easily available tests including blood sampling (lipids, glucose), urine dip, ECG and chest X-ray
> - A diagnostic test is chosen based on the pretest probability of coronary artery disease
> - Advanced investigations are individualised based on the patients and their specific clinical needs.

Treatment

Treatment is directed at reducing future risk of cardiovascular events and relieving symptoms.

Antiplatelet therapy

Although the beneficial effect of aspirin for secondary prevention following acute vascular events (including MI) has been unequivocally determined by clinical studies, the importance of aspirin in primary prevention has been debated. This is because, although aspirin does reduce vascular events, it is also associated with an increased risk of bleeding. The use of aspirin in this context should therefore be determined by a clinical assessment of the relative risk of vascular events versus bleeding.

Risk factor modification

Patients with stable angina should undergo optimal treatment of identified risk factors (Table 3.1).

Anti-anginal therapy

There are a number of effective anti-anginal therapies. For short-term-symptom relief, sublingual glycerine trinitrate (GTN) is effective and may be used prophylactically immediately before an activity likely to provoke angina. Beta blockade is recommended as first-line therapy. A cardioselective B-blocker may be selected where therapy is limited by mild reversible airways disease or peripheral vascular disease. The second-line therapy of choice is a calcium channel blocker. Other agents may be used in addition or as alternatives if use of a B-blocker and/or calcium channel blocker is limited by low heart rate and/or blood pressure. These include oral nitrates (note that a nitrate-free period overnight is required to prevent nitrate tolerance), nicorandil, ivabradine and ranolazine. These are particularly useful in refractory angina or where revascularisation is impossible.

Revascularisation

There are two techniques that can be used: percutaneous coronary intervention (PCI) or coronary artery bypass grafting (CABG).

PCI

This is an endovascular approach. A guiding catheter is sited in the coronary ostium (passed up from a percutaneous sheath usually placed in the radial or femoral artery). A fine wire is used to cross the coronary stenosis. This is used to pass coronary balloons that stretch the narrowed artery. Usually, a balloon expandable coronary stent is then deployed to scaffold the narrowing area and prevent arterial recoil. Drug-eluting stents may be used that elute antimitotic agents ablumenally to reduce the risk of localised neointimal proliferation and in-stent restenosis. To reduce the risk of stent thrombosis, a period of dual antiplatelet therapy with aspirin and clopidogrel is required after stenting. For bare metal stents, a period of 4 weeks is adequate. For drug-eluting stents, up to 12 months of therapy is required. A number of adjunctive technologies may be used to enhance PCI. These include intracoronary imaging [e.g. intravascular ultrasound (IVUS) and optical coherence tomography (OCT)] used to more clearly define coronary anatomy and measures of coronary physiology with pressure/flow wires [fractional flow reserve (FFR) and index of microcirculatory resistance (IMR)] used to differentiate flow-limiting stenoses requiring PCI from non-flow-limiting lesions that can be safely managed conservatively (Figure 3.4).

CABG

This requires open heart surgery and uses arterial or venous conduits to bypass proximal areas of disease by anastomosing grafts more distally to the epicardial coronary vessels. CABG (particularly where a left internal mammary artery LIMA graft is used) is associated with excellent long-term outcomes, provided patients are appropriately selected according to operative risk. The importance

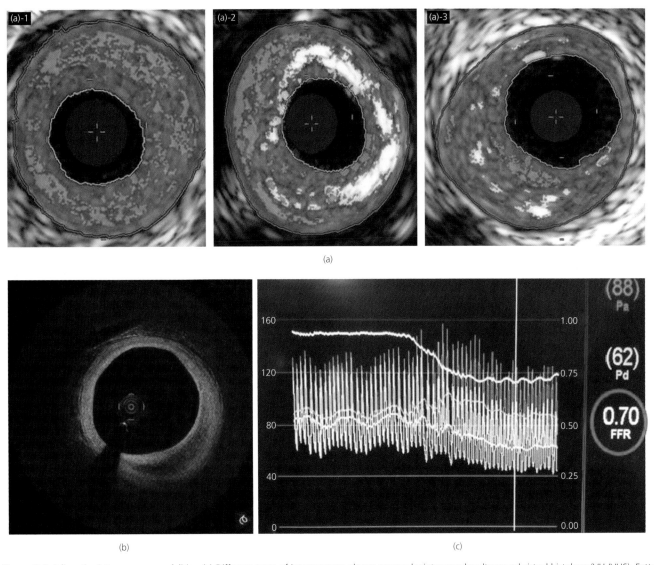

Figure 3.4 Adjunctive intracoronary modalities. (a) Different types of intracoronary plaque as seen by intravascular ultrasound virtual histology (VH-IVUS). Fatty tissue, fibro-fatty tissue, calcium and necrotic tissues are represented, respectively, by dark green, light green, white and red colours. (b) Optical coherence tomography (OCT) showing a large lipid plaque – bottom right of image. (c) Pressure wire assessment of a stenotic lesion showing a fractional flow reserve (FFR) of 0.70 (a significant FFR is <0.80).

of arterial grafting (in particular, the use of the right internal mammary artery) is subject of ongoing assessment in clinical trials.

CABG versus PCI for stable angina

Studies including COURAGE have demonstrated that there is no survival advantage in most patients with stable angina treated with PCI compared to those stabilised medically. In stable angina therefore revascularisation is usually reserved for patients with symptoms refractory to at least two anti-anginal medications or with a high ischaemic burden on functional imaging. Revascularisation may be undertaken by either PCI (usually with stenting) or coronary artery bypass surgery (CABG). The choice of revascularisation strategy is determined by the patient's operative risk and the location and extent of stenotic coronary disease (which can be calculated using the SYNTAX or similar scores). In general, CABG is favoured for patients with low operative risk and more extensive disease including significant left main stem or proximal three vessel disease.

Rare causes of angina

Aortic stenosis. when severe can lead to angina symptoms even in the absence of coronary restriction.

Microvascular angina. particularly in patients with diabetes or hypertensive heart disease, angina symptoms can arise from small vessel insufficiency without major epicardial coronary stenosis.

Coronary artery spasm. an exaggerated vasoconstrictor response can rarely cause symptomatic angina. Treatment is with vasodilators such as calcium channel blockers and avoidance of beta blockade.

Acute Coronary Syndrome (ACS)

Acute coronary syndromes (ACSs) are often divided into three clinical entities, unstable angina (UA) occurs when a patient presents with sudden onset angina, angina provoked by reducing levels of exercise or episodes of rest pain in the absence of biomarker evidence of myocardial necrosis. This is a clinical diagnosis. MI is usually divided by ECG criteria into ST-elevation myocardial infarction (STEMI) and non ST-elevation myocardial infarction (NSTEMI). Both are associated with elevations in circulating biomarkers of myocardial necrosis (such as troponin) STEMI is usually associated with thrombotic occlusion of a major epicardial coronary artery, whereas NSTEMI is more frequently a result of transient or incomplete occlusion, although the correlation between ECG and angiographic findings is by no means absolute.

This subdivision of ACS is clinically useful as it helps risk stratify patients. STEMI, in particular, is associated with high early risk of death that can be mitigated by prompt treatment and, in particular, immediate reperfusion.

Management of ACS
CCU care

ACS, and particularly STEMI and high-risk NSTEMI (such as those with ST-depression, pulmonary oedema and cardiogenic shock), is associated with early complications including malignant arrhythmias or ventricular fibrillation. This has led to the development of specialist high-dependency coronary care units in most hospitals. All patients presenting with ongoing symptoms require analgesia, usually with morphine (plus an antiemetic) and oxygen. Sublingual or intravenous nitrates can be considered if blood pressure is not limiting.

Dual antiplatelet therapy

All ACS benefit from early initiation of antiplatelet therapies. Aspirin is frequently administered in the community with a second therapy administered once the diagnosis has been confirmed. Current evidence favours the use of newer antiplatelet therapies (ticagrelor or prasugrel) over clopidogrel for ACS indications. Intravenous glycoprotein IIb/IIIa inhibitors may be used, although data for the role of these agents in the era of the newer oral therapies is awaited. Dual antiplatelet therapy should continue for 12 months following ACS unless a contraindication limits this. Aspirin should continue lifelong.

Immediate Revascularization in STEMI by Primary Percutaneous Intervention (PPCI)

All patients with ACS should be considered for angiography with a view to revascularisation. In those with STEMI, outcome is directly related to the time between symptom onset and restoration of flow in the occluded culprit coronary vessel. In most geographical areas, prompt coronary reperfusion in STEMI is achieved by primary percutaneous coronary intervention (PPCI) in which flow is restored by coronary thrombus aspiration, angioplasty and stenting (Figure 3.5). However, where timely access to PPCI is not practical, a strategy of out-of-hospital thrombolysis and transfer to a cardiac centre for early but not immediate angiography and stenting is also effective, provided there is no contraindication to thrombolysis (usually due to risk of bleeding).

Treatment of unstable angina and NSTEMI

Patients with UA or NSTEMI who do not have haemodynamic instability or dynamic ECG changes do not require immediate revascularisation but should have invasive angiography within 24–72 h of admission with a view to revascularisation (Figure 3.6). Otherwise, the approach to secondary prevention is the same (and just as important) as for STEMI. Indeed, although the immediate mortality from STEMI is higher, with modern reperfusion strategies, outcomes have significantly improved and

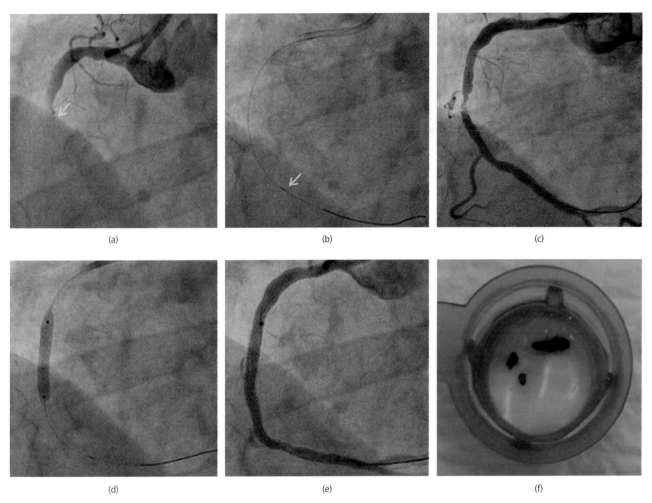

(a) (b) (c)

(d) (e) (f)

Figure 3.5 Primary angioplasty in a patient presenting with inferior STEMI. (a) Coronary angiogram showing completely occluded right coronary artery at mid vessel (arrow). (b) Angioplasty wire and thrombus aspiration catheter (arrow) in the vessel. (c) Some blood flow is restored after thrombus aspiration revealing a severe stenosis. (d) A stent is being deployed at the sight of stenosis. (e) Normal luminal diameter and blood flow restored with stent deployment. (f) Aspirated thrombus in a basket.

recent data has demonstrated major adverse cardiac events and mortality are higher in the medium and long term in patients with NSTEMI.

Secondary prevention

In addition to antiplatelet therapy, there are several key medical therapies that have been shown to improve long-term outcome. If possible, patients should be taking a high dose of a potent statin, an ACE inhibitor (or angiotensin receptor antagonist) and a beta-blocker. In addition, aldosterone receptor antagonists should be used in patients with impaired left ventricular systolic function post ACS. Hyperglycaemia should be managed acutely and longer term diabetic management optimised.

Cardiac rehabilitation programmes have a very important role in establishing an active and healthy life style and are very strongly recommended.

Rare causes of ACS

Spontaneous coronary dissection: This is rare condition with an increased incidence in young women, particularly in the peri- and post-partum period. A haematoma develops in the vessel wall leading to coronary restriction or occlusion.

Coronary artery embolus: Rarely cardiac or paradoxical emboli can enter the coronary circulation leading to ACS.

Coronary artery spasm: An exaggerated vasoconstriction can in extreme cases cause UA or even NSTEMI.

Takotsubo cardiomyopathy: A severe stress-induced coronary spasm causing ST elevation in ECG and leading to significant but mostly reversible left ventricular dysfunction. Angiography typically shows normal or insignificant coronary disease and antero-apical ballooning of the left ventricle.

Aortic dissection: Can occasionally cause ostial coronary restriction, particularly of the right coronary artery.

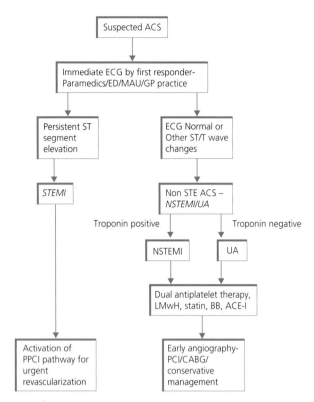

Figure 3.6 Flow diagram for management of acute coronary syndrome. ED, emergency department; MAU, medical assessment unit; STEMI, ST-elevation myocardial infarction; NSTE-ACS, non-ST elevation acute coronary syndrome; NSTEMI, non-ST elevation myocardial infarction; UA, unstable angina; PCI, percutaneous coronary intervention; CABG, coronary artery bypass graft surgery.

Acknowledgements

Dr. J. Baron for the CT Coronary Angiogram image and Dr. S. Hoole for the VH-IVUS image.

Clinical scenario: a 72-year-old man with acute anterior STEMI

Presentation: A 72-year-old man called 999 in the morning after developing severe, ongoing epigastric pain and some retrosternal discomfort after walking his dog. This was preceded by a 3-week history of milder and shorter lasting symptoms. He has a history of treated hypertension and hyperlipidaemia.

Assessment and management by paramedics: He looked clammy and sweaty and was in severe pain. An ECG showed ST elevation from

---

lead V1 to V5. He was given oral aspirin 300 mg, sublingual nitrate, IV morphine and antiemetic. The local PPCI pathway was activated and he was transferred directly to the cardiac catheter lab assessment area.

PPCI: Clinically, a diagnosis of anterior STEMI was made and he was taken into the cath lab for PPCI after consent was obtained. He received an oral loading dose of Prasugrel 60 mg. An urgent coronary angiogram was performed, which showed a completely occluded LAD (left anterior descending) proximally with no distal blood flow, and was successfully treated with deployment of a drug-eluting stent. This was achieved within 30 min of his hospital admission (target door to balloon/reperfusion time <90 min). His ECG normalised soon after and he was admitted to coronary care unit.

Further course and investigations: The patient had brief asymptomatic episodes of ventricular tachycardia that resolved within 24 h. He remained clinically well. His baseline blood results showed a highly sensitive Troponin T level of 900 ng/ml and a total cholesterol of 6.2 mmol/L. Bedside echocardiography showed only mild impairment of left ventricular systolic function.

Outcome: His medical therapy was titrated and he was discharged home on day 3 with routine follow-up and input from cardiac rehabilitation team.

Further reading

Armstrong WF and Zoghbi WA. Stress echocardiography: current methodology and clinical applications. *JACC* 2005;**45**(11):1739–1747.

Boden WE, O'Rourke RA, Teo KK *et al.* for the COURAGE Trial Research Group. Optimal medical therapy with or without PCI for stable coronary disease (The COURAGE trial), *N Engl J Med* 2007;**356**:1503–1516.

Conroy RM, Pyörälä K, Fitzgerald AP *et al.* Estimation of ten-year risk of fatal cardiovascular disease in Europe: the SCORE project. *Eur Heart J* 2003; **24**:987–1003.

ESC clinical Practice Guideline on Acute Coronary Syndromes (ACS) in patients presenting without persistent ST-segment elevation (Management of), 2011.

ESC clinical Practice Guideline on Acute Myocardial Infarction in patients presenting with ST-segment elevation (Management of), 2012.

Jahnke C, Nagel E, Ostendorf PC, *et al.* Diagnosis of a single coronary artery and determination of functional significance of concomitant coronary artery disease. *Circulation* 2006;**113**:e386–e387.

Libby P, Ridker PM and Hansson GK. Progress and challenges in translating the biology of atherosclerosis. *Nature* 2011;**473**:317–325.

NICE Guideline on chest pain of recent onset (CG95), 2010.

Sabharwal NK and Lahiri A. Role of myocardial perfusion imaging for risk stratification in suspected or known coronary artery disease. *Heart* 2003;**89**:1291–1297.

CHAPTER 4

Abdominal Aortic Aneurysms

David A. Sidloff, Nikesh Dattani, and Matthew J. Bown

Department of Cardiovascular Sciences, University of Leicester, UK

OVERVIEW

- Abdominal aortic aneurysms (AAAs) are an important cause of death, largely due to rupture. The epidemiology of AAA is changing with most developed countries noting a steady decline in AAA mortality over the last decade. Smoking is the most significant risk factor for AAAs and is the only modifiable risk factor that has been associated with the development, expansion and rupture of AAAs.

- The majority of AAAs are asymptomatic until the onset of complications, the most serious of which is rupture. The classical presenting triad of a ruptured AAA is pain, either abdominal or back pain, hypotension and a pulsatile abdominal mass. Other complications include the embolisation of thrombus from the AAA causing acute distal ischaemia and, less commonly, acute thrombosis.

- Clinical examination is not a reliable tool for the diagnosis of AAAs. The simplest diagnostic test for AAAs is ultrasound that has a sensitivity and specificity approaching 100%.

- AAA size is the single most important factor in determining the risk of rupture. Patients with large aneurysms (more than 5.5 cm) are usually offered surgery to prevent AAA rupture, provided they are fit enough. Elective aneurysm repair has a significantly lower peri-operative mortality (around 4%) than emergency repair of a ruptured AAA (around 40%).

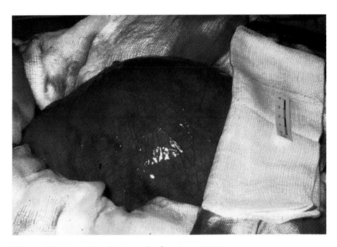

Figure 4.1 Operative photograph of an intact AAA.

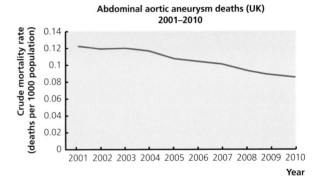

Figure 4.2 Death rates due to abdominal aortic aneurysm 2001–2010 in the United Kingdom. Data from the World Health Organisation mortality database (http://apps.who.int/healthinfo/statistics/mortality/whodpms/).

Introduction

The infra-renal abdominal aorta is the commonest site for arterial aneurysms, the vast majority of which are fusiform in shape (Figure 4.1). Abdominal aortic aneurysms (AAAs) cause approximately 4000 deaths per annum in England and Wales, largely due to rupture. The number of deaths due to AAAs rose throughout the 20th century; however, over the last decade, an unexplained, steady decline in AAA mortality has been noted in most developed countries (Figure 4.2). Despite this, the mortality rate following the rupture of AAAs in the community approaches 90%, making it an important cause of mortality. The true mortality of AAAs may even be higher as many patients dying from AAA rupture do not undergo formal post-mortem examination.

Definition

The true definition of aneurysmal arterial dilatation is an increase in vessel diameter of 50% or more in relation to an adjacent normal arterial segment. For practical purposes (in the case of the abdominal aorta), a measurement of greater than 3 cm in any axial diameter

ABC of Arterial and Venous Disease, Third Edition.
Edited by Tim England and Akhtar Nasim.
© 2015 John Wiley & Sons, Ltd. Published 2015 by John Wiley & Sons, Ltd.

is taken to be diagnostic for AAAs. Normal infra-renal diameter is 2.0–2.4 cm in males and 1.6–2.2 cm in females.

Epidemiology

In population screening studies of men over the age of 65, estimates for the prevalence of AAAs greater than 3 cm in size vary from 1.7% in the United Kingdom to 8.7% in New Zealand. The prevalence of AAAs is lower in women at approximately 1.5%. AAA is primarily a disease of white Europeans. They are extremely rare in Asian populations. This appears to be a genetic effect as Asian populations in the United Kingdom have a much lower incidence of AAAs than UK Caucasians. The incidence of AAAs also seems to be shifting towards an older population with males >75 years old now being the group most at risk.

Risk factors for abdominal aortic aneurysms (Box 4.1)

Smoking is the most significant risk factor for AAAs and is the only modifiable risk factor that has been associated with the development, expansion and rupture of AAAs. This has been confirmed by several prospective studies that have demonstrated a dose-dependent relationship and a 2.6 to 9.0 fold increase in risk of AAAs in smokers compared to non-smokers. The duration of smoking rather than amount smoked has a more significant effect on the risk of AAA formation and the risk of AAA only gradually reduces over time after smoking cessation.

Box 4.1 **Risk factors for AAAs**

Proven

- Tobacco smoking
- Age >60 years
- Gender (males)
- Genetics

Possible

- Hypertension
- Hyperlipidaemia
- Body mass index

Other risk factors have been identified for the formation of AAAs, although the strength of these associations is not as well defined as for smoking. Hypertension, hyperlipidaemia and an increased body mass index have all been associated with AAA development in some studies but other studies have failed to demonstrate this association. Interestingly, diabetes mellitus, which is traditionally a strong cardiovascular risk factor, seems to protect against both the development and the growth of AAAs.

Non-environmental risk factors for AAAs are age, race and gender. AAA rarely affects patients below the age of 40, and with increasing age, the prevalence of AAA increases. Above the age of 65, each 7-year age increment confers a 1.5-fold increase in the risk of AAAs. AAA is extremely rare in Asian populations and is

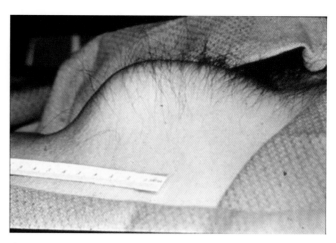

Figure 4.3 Photograph of a very thin patient with a large AAA that could be both seen and felt by the patient.

predominately a disease of males, the prevalence being nearly 6-fold greater in males than females. Although this sexual dimorphism exists among a number of cardiovascular diseases, it is not fully understood. There is a strong genetic component in the aetiology of AAAs, which appears to be due to multiple small-effect genetic loci rather than a single gene defect and studies to define the genetic risk factors for AAAs are ongoing.

Symptoms, signs and complications

The majority of AAAs (90%) are asymptomatic until the onset of complications, the most serious of which is rupture. Thin patients may notice a pulsatile swelling in their abdomen (Figure 4.3). The complications of any aneurysm are due to rupture, thrombosis or embolism. Acute thrombosis can occur in abdominal aneurysms but is more common in aneurysms at other sites such as the popliteal artery. Embolisation of thrombus from AAAs causing acute distal ischaemia (trash-foot) is more common than acute thrombosis (Figure 4.4). Together acute thrombosis or embolism only occur in 3–5% of patients with AAAs.

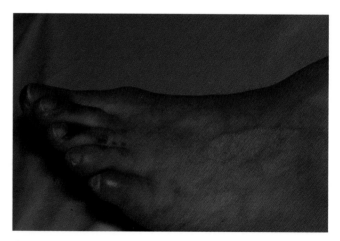

Figure 4.4 Focal infarction of areas of the first, second and third toes of the left foot in a patient with an AAA due to micro-embolisation of thrombus from within the aneurysm sac (trash-foot).

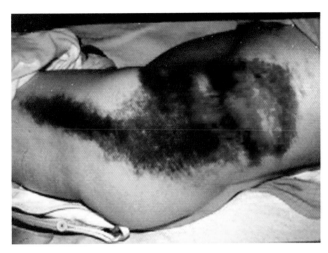

Figure 4.5 Flank bruising due to retroperitoneal blood from a ruptured AAA tracking laterally into the subcutaneous tissues. A rare sign of ruptured AAAs.

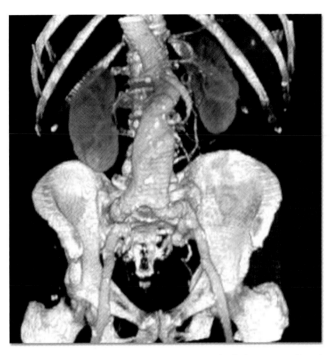

Figure 4.6 Three-dimensional computed tomography (CT) reconstruction of an infra-renal AAA. The kidneys and bony skeleton have been included in the reconstruction for reference.

The classical presenting triad of ruptured abdominal aortic aneurysms (RAAAs) is pain, either abdominal or back, hypotension and a pulsatile abdominal mass. As only approximately 25% of patients with RAAAs present with all the three signs, a high index of suspicion for RAAAs is essential in any patient who presents with any one of these symptoms and signs. Some patients may develop signs related to retroperitoneal haemorrhage such as flank or peri-umbilical bruising (Figure 4.5).

Diagnosis

Clinical examination is not a reliable tool for the diagnosis of AAAs. The simplest diagnostic test for AAAs is ultrasound that has a sensitivity and specificity approaching 100%. This also has the advantage of not requiring ionising radiation and because ultrasound technology is portable, it lends itself to being used as a community screening tool. Computerised tomography (CT) scanning has a similar sensitivity and specificity for the diagnosis of AAAs as ultrasound; however, CT also provides additional information regarding the morphology and anatomical relationships of the AAA (Figure 4.6). This information is essential in planning surgery and determining suitability for endovascular repair. Magnetic resonance imaging (MRI) provides similar information as CT but with the disadvantage of additional cost and limited patient acceptability. The main advantage of MRI is in the avoidance of ionising radiation.

In emergency situations, ultrasound scanning is useful to confirm the presence or absence of an AAA but cannot provide any information on the likelihood of AAA rupture. It is of most use in haemodynamically stable patients in whom the diagnosis of AAA is not suspected but needs to be excluded. CT scanning is more than 90% sensitive and specific for the detection of ruptured AAAs. Modern CT scanners can acquire images in as little as 30 s and thus cause little delay in transferring patients to theatre for surgery. The extra information provided and the possibility of assessment for endovascular repair are of significant benefit.

Risk of rupture

Before surgery for AAAs was developed in the second half of the 20th century, studies of patients with AAA who were left untreated demonstrated that 81.1% will die within 5 years compared to only 20.9% of the normal age-matched population. After 8 years, only 10% of those with AAA are alive compared to 65% of the normal population. In patients with AAA unfit for surgery, a quarter will die due to AAA rupture and the majority of these ruptures (80%) occur within 3 years of diagnosis.

AAA size is the single most important factor in determining the risk of rupture; however, rupture rates of small AAAs have been shown to be 2-fold higher in current smokers and 4-fold higher in women. Studies of ruptured AAAs have demonstrated that the median size is usually above 8 cm in diameter, whereas only a very small proportion of screening detected asymptomatic cases (0.16%) with greater than 6 cm in diameter. Autopsy studies have found that RAAAs are significantly larger than incidentally found intact AAAs (8 cm vs 4 cm). This implies that aneurysms are at higher risk of rupture as they increase in size.

Patients with large aneurysms (more than 5.5 cm) are usually offered surgery, provided they are fit enough. Patients with smaller aneurysms are a more difficult group to manage. Two large randomised controlled trials, one in the United Kingdom and one in the United States, have compared the strategy of early elective open surgical repair compared with surveillance in patients with small AAAs (4.0–5.5 cm). These studies demonstrated no survival advantage in patients undergoing early elective open surgery with similar findings after 12 years of follow-up in the UK Small Aneurysm Trial. Furthermore, the Comparison of Surveillance Versus Aortic Endografting for Small Aneurysm Repair (CAESAR) trial demonstrated similar findings with no advantage to early endovascular aneurysm repair (EVAR). Patients with asymptomatic AAAs that are less than 5.5 cm are, therefore, usually monitored ultrasonographically rather than offered surgery. Because of this relationship between size and risk of rupture, AAA size becomes the critical factor dictating clinical management.

Screening for AAAs

Screening programmes to detect AAAs have now been set up in many developed countries. The rationale behind AAA screening is that AAAs are often asymptomatic before rupture, have a long latent period and can be detected during an early phase in the disease using a test that is sufficiently sensitive, acceptable and cost effective. Furthermore, the mortality associated with AAA repair is significantly lower in the elective rather than emergency setting. The usefulness of AAA screening was first addressed in the Multicentre Aneurysm Screening Study (MASS) in 2002 that demonstrated a 42% risk of death reduction in a group of 65- to 74-year-old men screened for AAA. More recently, long-term data from this study suggests that the benefit of screening men aged 65–74 for AAA is maintained up to 13 years post screening and is highly cost effective in terms of cost per quality-adjusted life-year gained.

Surveillance

Following detection of a small AAA (<5.5 cm), patients are usually not offered surgery as the risks of surgery outweigh the current risk of rupture. However, because it is known that small AAAs grow with time, the risk of rupture also increases and it is important to provide surveillance for these patients. A recent meta-analysis of individual patient data by the RESCAN collaborators suggested that for each 0.5 cm increase in AAA diameter, growth rates increased on average by 0.59 mm per year and rupture rates increased by a factor of 1.91. A 3.5-cm AAA will on average take 6.2 years to reach 5.5 cm, whereas a 4.5 cm AAA will only take 2.3 years; therefore, the growth rate of AAAs is not linear. Currently, in the United Kingdom, those with 30–44 mm AAAs are offered yearly surveillance, whereas those with 45–54 mm AAAs are followed up every 3 months. In the future, patient-specific surveillance may become the standard of care.

Treatment

Currently, the only curative treatment for AAAs is surgery (Box 4.2). Traditionally, this consisted of open abdominal repair; however, since the early 1990s, endovascular techniques have become widely available and are rapidly advancing. While AAA is the main focus of this chapter, it should not be forgotten that each patient is likely to have significant cardiovascular risk factors and there is the opportunity to address these. Best medical therapy including antiplatelet agents, statins and antihypertensive medications in addition to smoking cessation advice should be considered in all patients. Improvements in the control of these common cardiovascular risk factors have likely contributed to the current decline in AAA-related mortality being observed in many developed economies.

Box 4.2 Outcome after AAA repair – peri-operative mortality rates

Elective surgery

Open repair	4.7%
Endovascular repair	1.2%

Emergency surgery for ruptured AAAs

Open repair	37.4%
Endovascular repair	35.4%

Elective AAA repair

Aside from AAA size, assessment of a patient's overall fitness, paying particular attention to cardio-respiratory and renal investigations, is important in any decision regarding suitability for surgery. A CT scan should also be obtained to determine the anatomy of the AAA and suitability for endovascular repair.

Open AAA repair consists of a laparotomy, isolation of the aneurysmal aorta between vascular clamps and after opening the aneurysm sac, suturing a synthetic graft in place and then closing the sac over the graft (an inlay repair) (Figure 4.7). This is a major procedure with an elective peri-operative mortality of 4.3% (from 3584 open repairs reported in the UK National Vascular Registry) and a risk of major systemic complications of approximately 25%. EVAR is an alternative to open AAA repair in those patients with anatomically suitable aneurysms. As EVAR has evolved, the boundaries of what is considered anatomically suitable have evolved with it (Figure 4.8). EVAR is much less invasive than open aneurysm repair, requiring only small femoral artery cut-down incisions rather than a full laparotomy. A suitably

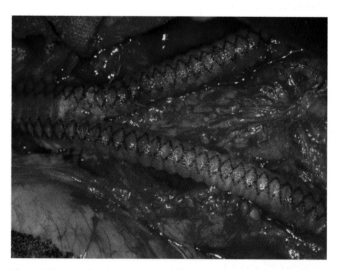

Figure 4.7 Operative photograph of a bifurcated Dacron graft inlay AAA repair. The proximal anastomosis lies to the left. The markings on the graft provide visual reference to prevent occlusion of the graft due to longitudinally twisting the graft during surgery.

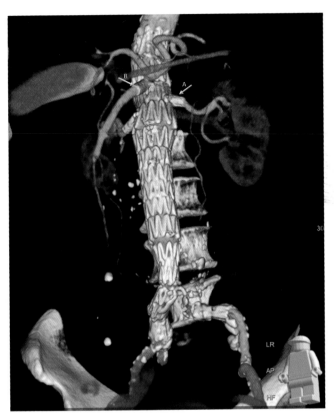

Figure 4.8 Three-dimensional CT reconstruction of an endograft used to repair an aneurysm. This endograft incorporates specially made fenestrations to allow the passage of blood into aortic side branches via secondary covered stents, for example, the left renal artery (A) and the superior mesenteric artery (B) in the treatment of para-renal AAA.

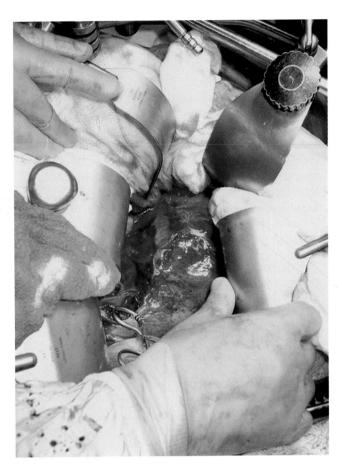

Figure 4.9 Operative photograph of a large retroperitoneal haematoma due to a ruptured AAA. The neck of the aneurysm is behind the haematoma at the top of the picture.

sized stent-graft is inserted via the femoral arteries and positioned in the infra-renal aorta under radiological guidance using specialised delivery systems. This procedure has been shown to have a 3-fold lower peri-operative mortality than open repair in large randomised trials (1.3% vs 4.7%) and in the United Kingdom has an overall elective mortality of 0.9% (from 4796 repairs). Of note, these mortality rates are significantly better than those reported only a few years ago and such improvements may be due to the centralisation of complex aortic surgery to high-volume centres in the United Kingdom as well as the instigation of the UK AAA Quality Improvement Programme.

This immediate survival advantage is offset by the requirement for life-long follow-up to detect potential complications that place the patient at continued risk of rupture including graft migration, graft material failure and leakage of blood around the graft into the AAA sac (endoleak). The peri-operative survival benefit seen in those receiving EVAR appears to be lost over time, which, in addition to EVAR carrying a significantly higher risk of reintervention and aneurysm rupture, makes any perceived advantage of EVAR over open AAA surgery less clear.

Ruptured AAA repair

The overall community mortality from ruptured AAAs is nearly 90%. In those patients who do reach hospital alive and undergo surgery (Figure 4.9), the peri-operative mortality is approximately 40%. Identifying those patients in whom surgery is futile is difficult. The most commonly used criteria predicting non-survival are extreme age (>80 years), pre-operative cardiac arrest, severe cardio-respiratory disease and unconsciousness. Endovascular techniques have been used with limited success in the treatment of ruptured AAAs; however, its place over open ruptured AAA repair is currently unclear. The IMPROVE trial randomised 613 patients with suspected ruptured AAAs, in 30 vascular centres, to undergo either EVAR or open repair (for patients anatomically unsuitable for EVAR). Endovascular repair was not associated with a significant reduction in either 30-day mortality or cost compared to open AAA repair; however, it did demonstrate the feasibility of endovascular repair for ruptured AAAs.

Clinical scenario: a patient with a leaking abdominal aortic aneurysm

Presentation: An 82-year old man presented to the casualty at around 3 AM with an episode of faint/collapse. Preceding this he had sudden onset of lower abdominal and back pain, a few hours earlier. He did not complain of any chest pain or shortness of breath. He also did not complain of any limb weakness. Before this he was fit and well, and on no regular medication. He was an ex-smoker and lived an independent, active life.

Examination findings: Alert and orientated, pulse rate 96/min (regular), BP 170/95, and oxygen saturation 96% (on air). Abdominal examination revealed a bit of distension and a tender mass around the umbilical region. The rest of the examination was unremarkable.

Differential diagnosis: (i) Leaking AAA, (ii) acute cardiac event, (iii) acute pancreatitis, (iv) other intra-abdominal pathology.

Investigations: (i) Blood tests (FBC, U&Es, glucose, clotting screen, lactate, amylase, Trop I and Cross-match), (ii) ECG (to exclude cardiac event), (iii) urgent abdominal CT scan.

Results: White cell count elevated, ECG showed sinus tachycardia and CT revealed contained rupture of a 10-cm-diameter AAA.

Management: Underwent laparotomy and repair of leaking AAA 1.5 h after presenting to casualty.

Outcome: Spent 5 days in ITU and discharged home 13 days post operation.

Further reading

Powell JT. Final 12-year follow-up of surgery versus surveillance in the UK Small Aneurysm Trial, The UK small aneurysm trial participants. *Br J Surg* 2007;**94**:702–708.

Powell JT on behalf of the IMPROVE trial investigators. Endovascular or open repair strategy for ruptured abdominal aortic aneurysm: 30 day outcomes from IMPROVE randomised trial. *Br Med J* 2014;**348**:f7661.

RESCAN Collaborators. Surveillance intervals for small abdominal aortic aneurysms: a meta-analysis. *J Am Med Assoc* 2013;**309**:806–813.

Thompson SG, Ashton HA, Gao L, *et al.* and on behalf of the Multicentre Aneurysm Screening Study (MASS) Group. Final follow-up of the Multicentre Aneurysm Screening Study (MASS) randomized trial of abdominal aortic aneurysm screening. *Br J Surg* 2012;**99**:1649–1656.

United Kingdom EVAR Trial Investigators, Greenhalgh RM, Brown LC, Powell JT, *et al.* Endovascular versus open repair of abdominal aortic aneurysm. *New Engl J Med* 2010;**362**:1863–1871.

CHAPTER 5

Visceral Artery Stenosis and Mesenteric Ischaemia

Daryll Baker

Department of Vascular Surgery, Royal Free Hospital, UK

OVERVIEW

- Visceral artery disease is caused by narrowing of the arteries that supply the intestines.
- It presents as two separate syndromes, acute mesenteric ischaemia (AMI) and chronic mesenteric ischaemia (CMI).
- AMI is a life-threatening vascular emergency that requires prompt diagnosis and treatment to prevent bowel necrosis and patient death.
- Diagnosis of both AMI and CMI remains a diagnostic challenge, because patients present with non-specific symptoms.
- Outcomes in both of these disorders can only be improved with rapid diagnosis and treatment that requires a high index of suspicion in patients presenting with abdominal pain who have multiple cardiovascular risk factors.

Introduction

Visceral artery disease is the narrowing of the arteries that supply blood to the intestines, spleen and liver. The visceral arteries are coeliac axis (CA), superior mesenteric artery (SMA) and inferior mesenteric artery (IMA). This disease process presents most commonly as two separate syndromes, acute mesenteric ischaemia (AMI) and chronic mesenteric ischaemia (CMI), although asymptomatic disease is common (20% of the older population) and chronic disease can present acutely.

Acute mesenteric ischaemia

Definition

AMI results from the sudden reduction in intestinal blood supply so severe as to result in bowel infarction.

Epidemiology

AMI occurs in 0.1% of hospital admissions, mainly in the older age group. It is associated with a greater than 70% mortality rising to 90% if bowel infarction has occurred. This can only be reduced with rapid vascular intervention, although the long-term prognosis remains grave with a 50% five-year survival rate.

Aetiology

Table 5.1 summarises the common causes of AMI. It arises primarily from problems in the SMA circulation or its venous outflow. Arterial disease may be due to occlusion of the SMA either from an embolus (50%) or from thrombosis of a pre-existing atherosclerotic lesion (25%). Arterial vasospasm can severely reduce mesenteric perfusion (20%) and mesenteric venous thrombosis can also cause bowel ischaemia (10%).

Table 5.1 Common causes of acute mesenteric ischaemia.

Mesenteric embolic causes

- Cardiac emboli

    Auricular thrombus associated with atrial fibrillation
    Mural thrombus after myocardial infarction
- Emboli from proximal aortic thrombus
- Emboli dislodged during arterial catheterisation

Thrombosis of pre-existing plaques

- Atherosclerotic vascular disease (most common)
- Aortic aneurysm
- Aortic dissection
- Arteritis

Mesenteric vasospasm

- Hypotension

    Cardiac failure
    Sepsis
    Severe liver or renal disease
- Vasopressor drugs
- Recent major cardiac or abdominal surgery

Mesenteric vein thrombosis

- Hypercoagulability states (congenital and acquired)
- Tumour causing venous compression
- Intra-abdominal infection
- Portal hypertension causing venous congestion
- Venous trauma

ABC of Arterial and Venous Disease, Third Edition.
Edited by Tim England and Akhtar Nasim.
© 2015 John Wiley & Sons, Ltd. Published 2015 by John Wiley & Sons, Ltd.

AMI does not include ischaemia caused by localised mechanical compression such as strangulated hernia, volvulus or intussusception.

Clinical presentation

The initial presentation of AMI is usually non-specific and diagnosis is therefore often missed initially, resulting in the significantly high mortality. A high clinical index of suspicion is vital in patients with the following presentation:

- Abdominal pain (95%). This is usually sudden and disproportionate to physical findings. Typically, the pain is moderate to severe, diffuse, non-localized and constant. It may be unresponsive to opiates, but peritonitic findings are often absent
- Gut emptying. Vomiting and diarrhoea (75%)
- Abdominal distension (25%)
- As the bowel becomes gangrenous, rectal bleeding and sepsis develops
- Clinical presentations that hint at an aetiology include:

  Atrial fibrillation or a recent myocardial infarction point to an embolic aetiology.

  Previous chronic mesenteric ischaemic symptoms (see the following sections) are present in 50% of patients with thrombotic AMI.

  Arterial vasospasm and mesenteric ischaemia tend to occur in older patients already unwell in the intensive care unit.

  In patients with mesenteric vein thrombosis, the abdominal pain tends to be less dramatic and can last for some weeks (30% have symptoms >30 days) and most have more than one risk factor for thromboembolic disease.

Investigations

Blood tests are not helpful in diagnosing AMI and tend to reflect developing bowel infarction, such that the white cell count and lactate levels are elevated and metabolic acidosis develops late in the clinical course. Elevated amylase levels are non-specific and phosphate levels are of no help.

If there is suspicion of AMI, radiographic studies should be undertaken without waiting for blood results. CT angiography is recommended as a first-line investigation as it has a greater than 90% sensitivity and specificity for diagnosing AMI. It will confirm the diagnosis and aid in planning treatment (Figure 5.1). Magnetic resonance angiography (MRA) yields findings similar to those of CT scanning in AMI (sensitivity of 100% and a specificity of 91%). It is particularly effective for evaluating mesenteric vein involvement. Therefore, it may be used in preference to CT depending on local radiological expertise. Plain abdominal X-rays and non-contrast CT help exclude other causes of the abdominal pain but identify AMI only when bowel infarction has developed. Duplex ultrasound is not usually performed in AMI as dilated loops of bowel reduce accuracy.

Treatment

Once the diagnosis is made, the treatment should be initiated without delay. The patient should have active resuscitation as per

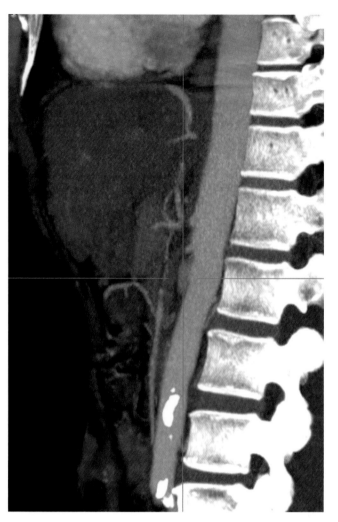

Figure 5.1 CT angiogram showing the aorta in front of the spine and occluded ostia of the mesenteric vessels.

hospital protocol for critically ill patients with a low threshold for involving the intensive care team. Intravenous fluid resuscitation with crystalloids and blood products should be started promptly to restore volume. Haemodynamic monitoring should be instituted with central venous pressure measurements and assessment of urinary output. Optimise cardiac status by treating any arrhythmia or congestive heart failure and providing inotropic support as required, but avoiding use of vasopressors. Ensure adequate tissue oxygenation by maintaining a saturation of over 95%, by endotracheal intubation and ventilation if necessary. The patient should receive adequate analgesia and intravenous broad-spectrum antibiotics should be commenced. Heparin anticoagulation is started as soon as the diagnosis has been made and before an urgent treatment plan has been determined. For venous AMI, this is often the only treatment required.

Revascularisation can be achieved by two methods: endovascular interventions or by open surgery involving a laparotomy.

Endovascular interventions are best undertaken in a hybrid operating theatre (Figure 5.2) in combination with open surgical procedures where potential complications (Table 5.2) can often be better managed. Thrombolytic agent infusion through

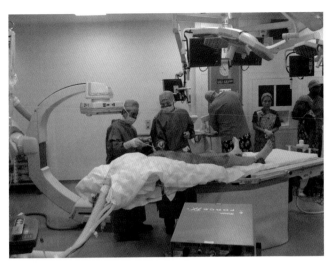

Figure 5.2 Complex vascular interventions are best done in a 'hybrid' theatre where both open and endovascular interventions can be performed.

Table 5.2 Potential complications of endovascular mesenteric revascularisation.

Dissection of mesenteric arteries
Rupture of mesenteric arteries. Small perforation can be covered
  with a stent graft, but larger ones require open surgery
Embolisation of atherosclerotic plaques causing bowel infarction
Groin haematoma
Acute limb ischaemia

an angiography catheter is considered when bowel infarction has not yet occurred. Bleeding is the main complication with use of thrombolysis. Angioplasty (after thrombolysis) with stent placement is indicated if the guide wire can cross the stenosis. Owing to the anatomy of the SMA, angioplasty and stenting

(Figure 5.3) are technically easier if a brachial approach is used. Suction embolectomy is not used as it often fails.

A laparoscopy may be perfumed to assess the viability of the bowel following a successful endovascular intervention. If there is evidence of irreversible bowel ischaemia, then a laparotomy is required to resect the necrotic bowel. Determination of bowel viability is difficult and the practice of viewing the bowel through a Wood lamp following fluorescein administration has not been universally adopted. Therefore, it is best to resect all areas of obviously necrotic bowel (Figure 5.4) and consider a 'second-look' laparotomy at 24–48 hours when the bowel has had sufficient time to recover and resected bowel ends can be anastomosed.

The open surgical approach involves performing an embolectomy to revascularise the ischaemic bowel. The SMA is isolated by palpating lateral to the aorta at the root of the lifted transverse colon mesentery, and because most emboli are near the origin of the middle colic artery, the pulse can be felt. A transverse arteriotomy is made proximal to the point of occlusion, and a balloon-tipped Fogarty catheter (size 3) passed distally. Often, a vein patch is needed to repair the arteriotomy. The small bowel should 'pink-up' within 10 minutes and a pulse felt or heard with the intra-operative Doppler machine. A bypass graft may be required if the bowel is not gangrenous and the cause is not embolic. An antegrade aorto-mesenteric bypass is performed using a reversed long saphenous vein (harvested from the upper thigh), as some form of faecal bacterial contamination is likely and insertion of a prosthetic risks infection.

Follow-up

Patients requiring extensive small bowel resection require follow-up by a gastroenterologist. Patients initially have severe diarrhoea but

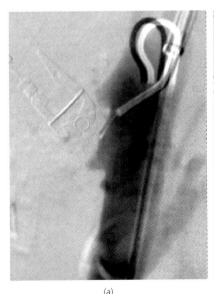

(a)

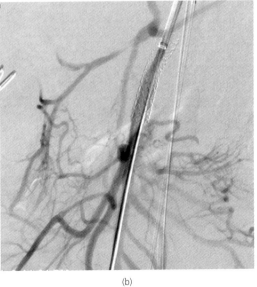

(b)

Figure 5.3 Endovascular management of a superior mesenteric artery occlusion. (a) Catheter angiogram demonstrating that all mesenteric vessels are occluded at the origin. (b) The superior mesenteric artery occlusion has been treated by angioplasty and stenting. A completion angiogram reveals good mesenteric blood supply.

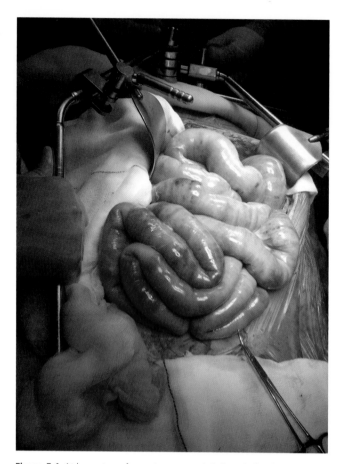

Figure 5.4 At laparotomy for acute mesenteric ischaemia (AMI), a bowel that is obviously infarcted needs to be resected. However, it is often difficult to determine the viability of the bowel as seen in this photo and a 'second-look' laparotomy should always be considered in such cases.

may be able to compensate after a few months with reduced loose bowel motions and begin to put on weight. Some patients have insufficient remnant small bowel and require total parenteral nutrition (TPN). The ileus secondary to intestinal ischaemia can cause adhesions and subsequent bowel obstruction. Patients who have had mesenteric vein thrombosis or are in atrial fibrillation will require warfarin therapy for life. Any cardiovascular risk factor should also be addressed in these patients.

Chronic mesenteric ischaemia (mesenteric angina)

Definition

The main symptom of CMI is mesenteric angina. This is significant postprandial pain that occurs due to extensive mesenteric vascular occlusive disease such that blood flow cannot increase enough to meet the visceral metabolic demands associated with digestion.

To produce such symptoms, at least two of the three mesenteric arteries need to be occluded as there is a vast network of collateral blood vessels linking them.

Epidemiology

The aetiology is almost always atherosclerotic stenotic disease. Those affected have multiple cardiovascular risk factors and atherosclerotic involvement of other territories such as coronary arteries, peripheral arterial disease and cerebrovascular disease. It is seen mainly in middle aged and elderly people and is three times more common in women. If not treated, the patient will suffer a painful death.

Clinical presentation

Patients classically complain of dull, postprandial epigastric pain, usually within the first hour after a meal. It gradually increases in intensity, reaches a plateau, and then slowly decreases in intensity several hours after eating. Initially, the pain develops only after large meals, but as the disease progresses, even small meals are poorly tolerated. The pain is out of proportion with the physical examination findings. Very commonly patients experience weight loss (80%) and often develop food aversion (sitophobia). Motility disturbances such as diarrhoea, bloating and vomiting can also be present. Physical examination reveals evidence of weight loss with signs of malnutrition and sometimes tenderness without rebound during episodes of pain. These patients may have bruits on auscultation of visceral arteries and also have reduced lower limb pulses.

Investigations

With these symptoms, a malignancy is often suspected that delays making the true diagnosis on average by 18 months. Blood tests do not help with making the diagnosis of CMI. They do, however, give an indication of the severity of the associated malnutrition. Duplex ultrasonography of the mesenteric vessels is a useful initial test in the clinic setting if the diagnosis is suspected. It is technically difficult but can be accomplished in around 85% of cases. CTA (or MRA) is recommended if duplex ultrasound is equivocal or for planning surgical intervention. In most cases, this will show that two of the three mesenteric vessels are occluded and the third is often severely stenosed. There will be an enlarged 'meandering' mesenteric marginal artery (of Drummond) acting as a collateral supply. Catheter-based angiography is indicated only during endovascular intervention.

Treatment

The indication for treatment is symptoms associated with mesenteric vessel occlusions. Asymptomatic lesions are not treated. There is no effective medical treatment but patients benefit from being on antiplatelet and statin therapy to reduce their long-term cardiovascular risk. Intervention for CMI is urgent rather than emergency and, therefore, can be planned and the patient's cardiovascular co-morbidities optimised. TPN feeding while this is being undertaken will help counter some of the peri-operative detrimental effects of malnutrition. Revascularisation of the gut is by either endovascular or open surgical techniques.

Endovascular surgical interventions are best undertaken in a hybrid theatre (Figure 5.2) under general anaesthetic as the potential complications may require open surgery (Table 5.2).

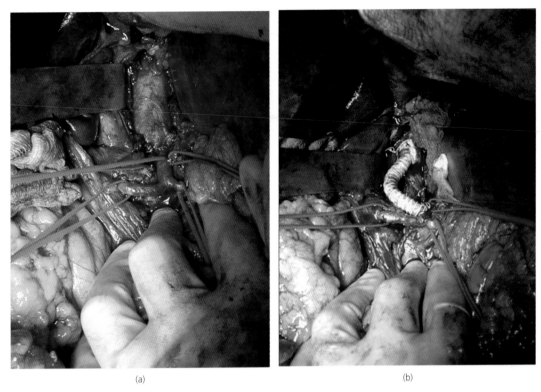

(a)   (b)

Figure 5.5 A laparotomy has been performed to deal with an occluded coeliac artery. (a) Coeliac artery and its early branches have been exposed. (b) A synthetic jump bypass graft has been performed from the aorta to the celiac artery past the occlusion.

Vascular surgical intervention options include

- bypass jump grafting, using either a vein or a prosthetic graft (Figure 5.5), and
- endarterectomy – surgical removal of the plaque.

It is usual practice to try and revascularise at least two of the three vessels. Treatment approach adopted will depend on the local facilities and expertise, as well as the general health of the patient and their associated co-morbidities. Compared to open surgery, an endovascular approach is considered to be less invasive with lower intra-operative mortality rates (6% versus 12%) and is associated with a shorter hospital stay (3 days versus 12 days), but with a lower long-term durability (30% versus 66% 3-year symptom-free outcome).

Follow-up

Patients who survive surgical revascularisation tend to do well, with excellent long-term prognosis (5-year survival rates approach 80%). Regular follow-up review includes duplex ultrasound and MRI (rather than CTA to reduce radiation exposure) to assess for re-stenosis. However, as the proper management of asymptomatic re-stenosis is unclear, further intervention should only be considered with the recurrence of symptoms, thus achieving an 80% 5-year symptom-free rate.

Conclusions

Symptomatic mesenteric ischaemia is a relatively rare but a potentially life-threatening disorder with very poor outcomes. An early diagnosis remains the key challenge in both AMI and CMI and requires a high index of suspicion in patients presenting with abdominal pain who have significant cardiac disease or multiple cardiovascular risk factors. Outcomes in this condition can only be improved by rapid diagnosis and treatment.

Clinical scenario: a patient with chronic mesenteric ischaemia

Presentation: An 80-year-old man was referred by a gastroenterologist after suspicion of mesenteric vascular disease on CT scan. He gave a 12-month history of postprandial abdominal pain associated with 3 stone weight loss. He had undergone extensive gastrointestinal tract investigations (including endoscopies) to look for a cause such as peptic ulceration or malignancy. He had history of IHD (ischaemic heart disease), hypertension and was a current smoker.

Examination findings: Patient was of a thin build with a soft non-tender abdomen. On auscultation, he had an audible bruit over the abdominal aorta. He had absent lower limb pulses suggestive of chronic peripheral vascular disease.

Differential diagnosis: Peptic ulcer disease, GI tract malignancy, mesenteric angina, chronic pancreatitis.

Investigations: Blood tests (FBC, U&Es, LFTs, cholesterol, glucose), CT/MR angiogram.

Results: Blood tests revealed mild anaemia (Hb 10.6 g/dl) and chronic renal impairment (eGFR 56 ml/min). His CT angiogram revealed atherosclerotic disease in the abdominal aorta with occlusion at origin of both coeliac and inferior mesenteric arteries. There was also a tight stenosis at the origin of the SMA.

Management: He was already on aspirin and statin therapy for IHD. In view of the above-mentioned symptoms, he underwent successful angioplasty and stenting of the SMA stenosis. His postprandial abdominal pain resolved immediately after the procedure. At 3-month follow-up, he was symptom free and had gained 1 stone in weight.

Further reading

Chang RW, Chang JB, Longo WE. Update in management of mesenteric ischaemia. *World J Gastroenterol* 2006;**12**(200):3243–3247.

Pecoraro F, Rancic Z, Lachat M, *et al.*. Chronic mesenteric ischemia: critical review and guidelines for management. *Ann Vasc Surg* 2013;**27**(1):113–122.

Fung K, Dawson J. Clinical review – mesenteric ischaemia. http://www.gponline.com/Clinical/article/1110549/clinical-review-mesenteric-ischaemia/ (accessed 17 March 2014).

Oldenburg WA, Lau LL, Rodenberg TJ, *et al.* Acute mesenteric ischemia: a clinical review. *Arch Intern Med* 2004;**164**(10):1054–1062.

CHAPTER 6

Acute Limb Ischaemia

Christos D. Karkos and Thomas E. Kalogirou

5th Department of Surgery, Medical School, Aristotle University of Thessaloniki, Hippocratio Hospital, Greece

OVERVIEW

- Acute limb ischaemia is a vascular surgical emergency that carries a high morbidity and mortality.
- Complete arterial ischaemia leads to tissue necrosis and the need for amputation within 6–12 h unless reperfusion occurs.
- Loss of motor function in the calf and foot muscles is an indication for immediate revascularisation.
- Thrombolysis will often unmask the underlying lesion that triggered thrombosis and permit subsequent correction by a percutaneous intervention or open surgery.
- Calf swelling and pain out of proportion following reperfusion of an ischaemic limb indicates compartment syndrome that should be relieved by emergency fasciotomy.

Introduction

Acute limb ischaemia (ALI) is defined as a sudden decrease in limb perfusion that causes a potential threat to limb viability (manifested by ischaemic rest pain, ulcers and/or gangrene) in patients who present within 2 weeks of the acute event. It is one of the most common emergencies in vascular surgery affecting about 14–16 per 100 000 inhabitants annually. The incidence increases with age and it is seen with equal frequency in men and women. A vascular unit serving a community of half a million can expect to treat approximately 75 such patients each year.

Clinical features

The 'six P's' have been used as a mnemonic to remember the presentation of a patient with ALI (Table 6.1). However, in daily practice, not all of these will necessarily be present in all patients. A subtle clinical picture is not uncommon, reflecting an adequate collateral supply (due to pre-existing atherosclerosis) and the often incomplete nature of the occlusion.

Pain: It is the most common symptom in ALI and is often severe, continuous and localised in the foot and toes. Its intensity does not reflect the severity of ischaemia. In less severe cases, it may be

Table 6.1 The six P's: symptoms and signs of ALI.

History (three P's)
- Pain
- Paraesthesia
- Paralysis

Clinical examination (three P's)
- Pallor
- Pulselessness
- Perishing cold (other authors include 'poikilothermia' as the sixth P, i.e. the limb may take on the ambient temperature)

absent, while in more severe cases, it may decrease with improving collateral perfusion or because sensory loss interferes with perception. Diabetic patients often have a degree of neuropathy and a decreased sensation of pain.

Paraesthesia: It starts as a feeling of numbness and soon progresses to loss of sensation to light touch. This is because thin nerve fibres conducting impulses from light touch are very sensitive to ischaemia and are damaged soon after perfusion is interrupted. In contrast, with pain fibres being less ischaemia-sensitive, finding a decreased pain perception indicates a much later stage of ischaemia.

Paralysis: It can be due to ischaemic damage of either the motor nerves or the muscle itself. In cases of severe proximal ischaemia, the entire limb can become paretic, which may be misinterpreted for a stroke. The inability to dorsiflex and plantarflex the toes is an ominous sign indicating impending necrosis of calf muscles and should prompt immediate revascularisation. Development of firm, spastic musculature (rigour), especially if the contralateral side is normal, indicates extensive muscle necrosis. Attempts to revascularise such a limb are futile.

Pallor: Initially, the acutely ischaemic limb is pale ('marble' white) due to arterial spasm, but over the next few hours, secondary vasodilatation occurs and blotchy mottled areas of cyanosis develop (representing areas of stagnant blood flow). Failure of the blue blotches to blanch on pressure (fixed mottling) is a sign of capillary bed thrombosis, indicating irreversible ischaemia (Figure 6.1).

Pulselessness: In general, palpable peripheral pulses exclude severe ischaemia, whereas sudden loss of a previously palpable pulse indicates acute arterial occlusion. Although the prior pulse

ABC of Arterial and Venous Disease, Third Edition.
Edited by Tim England and Akhtar Nasim.
© 2015 John Wiley & Sons, Ltd. Published 2015 by John Wiley & Sons, Ltd.

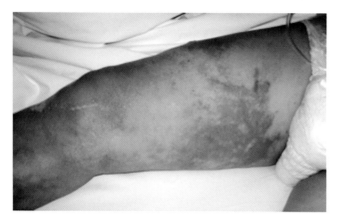

Figure 6.1 Fixed mottling extending up to the level of the upper thigh and is indicative of irreversible ischaemia and tissue necrosis.

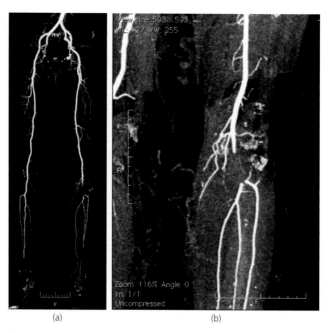

(a)   (b)

Figure 6.2 Computed tomography angiogram (CTA) of a patient with a popliteal artery embolus. (a) The entire arterial tree of both lower limbs looks normal, apart from an abrupt cut-off (filling defect) in the left below-the-knee popliteal artery, which is in keeping with the diagnosis of embolism. (b) The embolus lodged at the point where the artery bifurcates into the anterior tibial artery and the tibioperoneal trunk.

status of the limb is unlikely to be known, in most cases, the diagnosis can be facilitated by comparing the presence of pulses in the opposite limb.

Perishing cold: Examination will also reveal coldness of the limb about one joint distal to the level of obstruction. The point of occlusion, therefore, can be estimated by the level where the colour and temperature change and the pulse disappears.

The severity of ALI at initial presentation determines the limb outcome and is classified into three categories (Table 6.2).

Aetiology

The major causes of ALI are (i) embolism, (ii) thrombosis, (iii) occlusion of a vascular graft and (iv) trauma.

Embolism

Embolic causes were historically the most common, but with the diminishing prevalence of rheumatic heart disease, they are nowadays responsible for <30–40% of cases. Emboli originate from a proximal source (e.g. the heart or an aneurysm) and lodge at the points of arterial bifurcation, where the vessel diameter decreases abruptly (Figure 6.2), or at points of significant arterial stenoses (in cases of concurrent occlusive disease). The lower limb arteries are affected about five to six times as frequently as those of the upper limb. Embolism usually occurs in the setting of atrial fibrillation or

acute myocardial infarction, but other less common cardiac sources also exist (Table 6.3). Frequent non-cardiac causes include peripheral aneurysms or ulcerated atherosclerotic plaques.

Cholesterol embolisation (atheroembolism) is a particular form of embolism, in which a portion of the plaque breaks off and undergoes embolization to smaller diameter peripheral arteries, such as the digital arteries. In the latter case, one may be faced with the paradox of a patient who has ischaemic toes (or fingers) but palpable distal pulses. This condition is known as *trash foot* or *blue toe syndrome* and may occur spontaneously or follow diagnostic or therapeutic procedures, vascular or cardiac surgery. A similar situation can be seen with popliteal (or other peripheral) aneurysms. Occasionally, a cervical rib may compress the subclavian artery (thoracic outlet syndrome), resulting in a post-stenotic dilatation or aneurysm immediately distal to an area of compression and cause emboli in the hand (blue finger).

Table 6.2 Rutherford categories of ALI based on clinical findings and Doppler signals.

Category	Description and prognosis	Findings		Doppler signals	
		Muscle weakness	Sensory loss	Arterial	Venous
(I) Viable	Not immediately threatened	None	None	Audible (>30 mmHg)	Audible
(IIa) Marginally threatened	Salvageable if promptly treated	None	Minimal (toes) or none	Inaudible	Audible
(IIb) Immediately threatened	Salvageable with immediate revascularisation	Mild, moderate	More than toes, associated with rest pain	Inaudible	Audible
(III) Irreversible	Major tissue loss or permanent tissue damage inevitable	Profound paralysis	Profound, anaesthetic	Inaudible	Inaudible

Table 6.3 Causes of embolic occlusion.

Cardiac causes

Most common:
- atrial fibrillation (32–75%)
- myocardial infarction with mural thrombi (21–32%)

Less common:
- idiopathic dilated cardiomyopathy
- prosthetic valves
- endocarditis (bacterial or fungal)
- rheumatic mitral valve disease
- cardiac tumours, e.g. atrial myxomas (rare)
- paradoxical embolism (usually through a patent foramen ovale)

Non-cardiac causes
- Peripheral aneurysms (aortic, popliteal, iliac, femoral, subclavian, axillary) (5%)
- Ulcerated atherosclerotic plaques ('penetrating atherosclerotic ulcer' usually located in the descending thoracic aorta)

Unknown

Thrombosis

Thrombotic occlusion of native arteries is nowadays the commonest cause of ALI. Thrombosis, as an aetiology for ALI, is a much more diverse category than embolism (Table 6.4). Arterial thrombosis most often develops at the points of severe stenosis, typically of the superficial femoral or popliteal artery. However, a thrombus can be formed in the absence of significant pre-existing stenosis, particularly when the surface of the plaque is ulcerated or after an intraplaque haemorrhage resulting in sudden arterial occlusion. Popliteal aneurysms may also thrombose acutely, a condition that is associated with a high risk of limb loss due to the propagation of thrombus into the crural vessels (Figure 6.3). Other factors leading to thrombosis of a diseased artery (or even of a relatively normal one) are low-flow or hypercoagulable conditions. When faced with a young patient without atherosclerotic risk factors who

Table 6.4 Thrombotic causes of ALI.

Atherosclerotic disease

Popliteal and other less common peripheral arterial aneurysms

Low-flow conditions (e.g. cardiac failure, immobility, hypovolaemia, hypotension of any cause or decreased blood flow due to a more proximal stenosis)

Hypercoagulable states (e.g. myeloproliferative disorders, hyperviscosity syndromes and coagulation disorders)

Aortic dissection

Fibromuscular dysplasia (occasionally involving the iliac arteries)

Cystic adventitial disease (usually affecting the popliteal artery)

Thoracic outlet syndrome

Popliteal entrapment syndrome

Arteritides (e.g. Takayasu's aortitis and giant cell arteritis)

Thromboangiitis obliterans (involving medium-sized muscular arteries)

Compartment syndrome

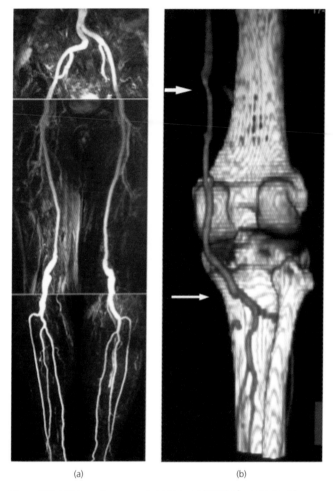

(a)　　　　　　　　　　(b)

Figure 6.3 (a) Magnetic resonance angiogram (MRA) of a patient with bilateral popliteal artery aneurysms. (b) Post-operative CTA of another patient who presented with ALI due to a thrombosed right popliteal aneurysm and underwent open surgical repair by means of distal thrombectomy, on-table thrombolysis and interposition bypass with reversed long saphenous vein (white arrows).

presents with ALI, the presence of malignancy, hyperviscosity and prothrombotic syndromes should be considered as possible causes, along with anatomical rarities, such as popliteal entrapment or thoracic outlet syndrome.

Graft occlusion

Prosthetic and venous bypass grafts may occlude for a variety of reasons. Early failures (within the first month) are usually due to technical problems at the time of surgery or poor run-off. Medium-term failures (occurring at around 1 year) are due to intimal hyperplasia at the anastomoses. Vein graft occlusion may also be caused by the development of stenosis within the graft itself (e.g. retained valve cusp of an *in situ* vein graft or the site of pervious thrombophlebitis). Late failures are usually caused by progression of proximal or distal atherosclerosis.

Trauma

Arterial trauma (either blunt or penetrating) is a common cause of ALI. Possible mechanisms include artery transection, intimal disruption or spasm due to a large expanding haematoma.

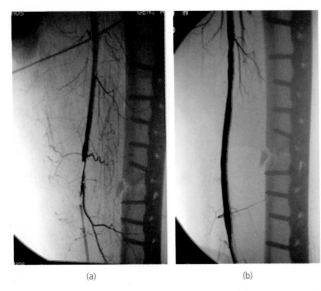

(a)   (b)

Figure 6.4 (a) Intimal disruption of the superficial femoral artery as a result of a femoral shaft fracture. (b) The patient was successfully treated by balloon angioplasty and stent placement.

Acute traumatic limb ischaemia may also result from limb fractures and dislocations (Figure 6.4) or be iatrogenic (e.g. percutaneous cardiology and vascular interventions, vascular and orthopaedic limb surgery, general surgical, gynaecological or urological procedures in the pelvis).

Management and treatment

Distinguishing embolism from thrombosis, although not always feasible, is desirable because treatment is different (Table 6.5). However, it is the severity of ischaemia that should largely dictate the management. Muscle paralysis, tense swollen fascial compartments and fixed skin staining (i.e. Rutherford category III) characterise the irreversible limb ischaemia, which is, by definition, an indication for primary amputation after appropriate resuscitation and stabilization of the patient. The prevention of limb loss in the Rutherford IIb category (acute white leg with sensorimotor deficit) requires immediate intervention. On the other hand, moderate ALI with acute onset of rest pain with no concomitant paralysis and only mild sensory loss (i.e. Rutherford IIa category) represents the majority of the patients and is often due to acute thrombosis of an atherosclerotic segment. As the limb is not immediately threatened, there is time to plan appropriate intervention with arteriography.

Table 6.5 History and clinical findings pointing towards an embolic cause for ALI.

Acute onset where the patient is often able to accurately time the moment of the event

Prior history of embolism

Known embolic source (such as cardiac arrhythmias)

No prior history of intermittent claudication

Normal pulse and Doppler examination in the unaffected limb

General measures – conservative treatment

ALI is often the tip of the iceberg of a patient in poor clinical condition with multiple co-morbidities. Many patients suffer from dehydration, cardiac failure, hypoxia and pain that should be managed in the standard way. Urgent venous access, pain relief, oxygen, rehydration and intravenously given heparin (5000 units) may help in stabilizing the patient and limit propagation of thrombus.

Surgery

When an embolus is suspected, embolectomy with a balloon catheter is performed under local anaesthesia (Figure 6.5). Standard embolectomy is usually performed blind (i.e. there is no control over the direction of the catheter past the popliteal trifurcation), and as a result, residual thrombus may well be left behind. An alternative is to use an over-the-wire catheter that can be selectively guided to each one of the crural arteries under fluoroscopy. On completion of the procedure, an on-table angiogram can be performed to check the result. If the initial procedure is unsatisfactory, further options are exposure and direct embolectomy of the popliteal and distal arteries, bypass or on-table thrombolysis.

Contrary to embolism, arterial thrombosis is unlikely to be effectively treated by balloon catheter thrombectomy alone. Provided that ischaemia is not absolute (which is usually the case in most patients with thrombosis due to pre-existing disease), there is time for preoperative angiography. A wider variety of options are available in these patients, including open surgery (endarterectomy, bypass), endovascular interventions (balloon angioplasty, stenting) or thrombolysis.

Thrombolysis

Thrombolysis for ALI is best achieved via a percutaneous, catheter-directed, intra-arterial technique. Recombinant tissue plasminogen activator (rtPA) and urokinase are currently the most commonly used thrombolytic agents, whereas streptokinase is less popular because of fear of allergic reactions. Compared to surgery, thrombolysis is generally less invasive and can open both large and small vessels (the latter being inaccessible to surgical thrombectomy or bypass). It may be used as a monotherapy, i.e. obviating the need for surgery, or it may convert a major emergency operation to an elective one of a lesser magnitude. By dissolving the thrombus, thrombolysis will often unmask the underlying, flow-limiting lesion that triggered thrombosis and permit subsequent correction by the most appropriate percutaneous or open surgical technique. However, it cannot be used in patients with complete ischaemia because thrombus dissolution takes several hours and permanent muscle death follows 6–12 h of ischaemia. Such patients should undergo emergency revascularisation. Even so, thrombolysis may still be used in these cases as an adjunct to clear run-off vessels. There are several contraindications to thrombolysis, so one should be careful in patient selection (Table 6.6). Because of the risk of bleeding and systemic complications (minor haemorrhage 20–40%, major haemorrhage 5–10%, stroke 3%), and also because the ischaemic leg may deteriorate, careful monitoring during thrombolysis is necessary. This is best done in an intensive care or step-down unit by experienced nursing and medical staff. Clinical deterioration during thrombolysis signals the need to interrupt the infusion and

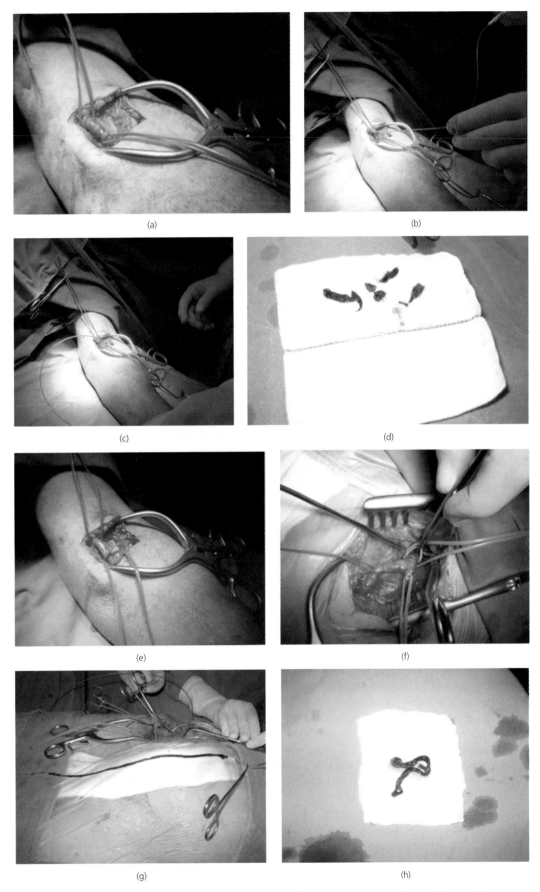

Figure 6.5 Balloon catheter embolectomy. In the upper limb, an antecubital fossa incision is made to expose the brachial artery (a), a transverse arteriotomy is performed, the balloon catheter (known as *Fogarty catheter*) is passed both proximally (b) and distally (c) until two successive passes yield no further clots (d) and the arteriotomy is repaired (e). In the lower limb, a vertical groin incision is made to expose the femoral bifurcation and the arteries are controlled with silastic slings (f). Here, the entire column of the propagated thrombus has been removed intact from the superficial femoral artery (g, h).

Table 6.6 Contraindications for thrombolysis in ALI.

Active internal bleeding (absolute)

Intolerable ischaemia

Cerebrovascular accident within 2 months

Intracranial pathology (known intracerebral tumour, aneurysm or
  arteriovenous malformations)

Craniotomy within 2 months

Transient ischaemic attack within 2 weeks

Recent major surgery or trauma (<10 days)

Vascular surgery within 2 weeks

Previous gastrointestinal tract bleeding

Severe hypertension

Coagulation disorders

Pregnancy

Recent eye surgery or diabetic retinopathy

Puncture of a non-compressible vessel or biopsy within 10 days

Severe liver disease

Severe renal failure

proceed with surgical revascularisation. New developments, on the other hand, such as mechanical or aspiration thrombectomy, may enhance the effectiveness of thrombolysis, particularly, in cases of high bulk of initial thrombus or where the initial thrombolysis fails (high amount of residual thrombus).

Several randomised trials and a recent Cochrane review concluded that there is no difference in limb salvage or death at 1 year, and, therefore, universal initial treatment with either surgery or thrombolysis cannot be advocated on the available evidence. Thrombolysis may be associated with a higher risk of ongoing limb ischaemia and haemorrhagic complications, but this higher risk of complications must be balanced against the risks of surgery in each person. The final choice would depend on local policy, preference and expertise.

Ischaemia–reperfusion

Patients treated for severe ALI are at risk of developing ischaemia–reperfusion syndrome, a condition that can be more harmful than ischaemia alone. When perfusion of ischaemic muscles is restored, metabolites from damaged and disintegrated muscle cells are spread systemically and may cause further tissue injury both locally (manifested as compartment syndrome) and at remote sites. Oxygen free radicals and neutrophil activation play an important role in this complex process. Systemic manifestations may include acute renal failure (metabolic acidosis, hyperkalaemia, myoglobinuria, and acute tubular necrosis), myocardial depression (cardiogenic shock, arrhythmias, infarction and cardiac arrest), acute respiratory distress syndrome (ARDS), hepatic failure or gastrointestinal endothelial oedema leading to increased gastrointestinal vascular permeability and endotoxic shock. The elevated mortality encountered in severe ALI may be due to the above-mentioned complications and avoiding or minimising the effects of reperfusion may improve survival. Candidates at significant risk for reperfusion are those with longer ischaemia times (>4–6 h) and

those with more proximal occlusions (e.g. saddle emboli in the aortic bifurcation) where the affected muscle mass is large. Treatment includes correction of underlying abnormalities, such as acidosis and hyperkalaemia, hydration and maintaining a good urine output, alkalinisation of the urine with sodium bicarbonate, mannitol (acting both as an osmotic agent to induce diuresis and a scavenger of deleterious oxygen free radicals) and, in some cases, haemodialysis. Cardiorespiratory support may also be required in certain patients.

Compartment syndrome

The acute inflammation in the muscle after restoring perfusion leads to swelling and, as the available space for the muscles within the confined fascial compartment is limited, the increased pressure in the compartments reduces capillary blood perfusion below the level necessary for tissue viability (compartment syndrome). As a result, nerve injury and muscle necrosis can occur. The amount of oedema parallels the severity and duration of the ischaemia. The main clinical feature is pain – often very strong and 'out of proportion' – which is accentuated by squeezing the calf or passive dorsiflexion of the foot. Pedal pulses may still be present and do not exclude the syndrome. Treatment consists of emergency fasciotomy (Figure 6.6).

Post-operative anticoagulation

Following embolectomy, patients with atrial fibrillation should be on long-term anticoagulation with warfarin to reduce the risk

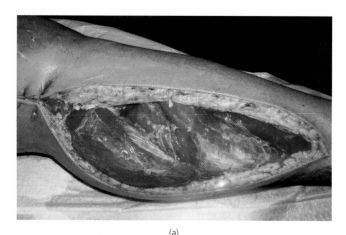

(a)

(b)

Figure 6.6 Fasciotomy for compartment syndrome. Decompression of all four compartments of the leg has been achieved using two long incisions, one placed laterally (not seen here) and one medially in the calf (a). The wounds can be closed or skin-grafted later (b).

of recurrent embolism. When non-cardiac causes of embolism (such an aneurysm or a penetrating aortic ulcer) are identified, these should be treated accordingly. If the source of the emboli is not clear, it should be investigated. If no source of embolism is found (which is the case in 5–12% of patients despite a full diagnostic work-up), anticoagulation should continue long term. Long-term anticoagulation should also be considered in cases of arterial thrombosis when the risk of recurrent thrombosis persists.

Prognosis

The outlook for patients admitted with ALI has generally been poor. Only 60–70% of patients leave the hospital with an intact limb. The 30-day mortality is 15–30% and 15% of the survivors undergo an amputation. Mortality is higher in patients presenting with embolic causes (due to the underlying cardiac disease), whereas limb loss is higher in those with thrombosis. Long-term outcome is equally poor with only 30–40% of the patients being alive at 5 years (probably due to a combination of advanced age and co-morbidities).

Clinical scenario: a patient with acute limb ischaemia

Presentation: A 78-year-old female with known insulin-dependent diabetes mellitus, atrial fibrillation (but not on warfarin) and heart failure presented with a 6-h history of acute onset pain in her right leg associated with paraesthesia of the foot.

Examination findings: She had a pale, cold right foot with mild sensory and motor deficit. There was no tenderness of the calf muscles. She had absent pulses from the femoral artery down on the right side. The left leg had full complement of pulses.

Differential diagnosis: Acute limb ischaemia secondary to an embolus, acute cardiac event with poor peripheral perfusion, acute on chronic arterial ischaemia, nerve root compression, ruptured Baker's cyst.

Investigations: Blood tests and ECG. The diagnosis is essentially clinical and imaging only delays the treatment (and increases risks of complications from prolonged limb ischaemia). Imaging should only be performed at the discretion of a vascular surgeon.

Management: A clinical diagnosis of acute limb ischaemia secondary to thromboembolism was made and the patient taken immediately to the operating theatre for femoral embolectomy under local anaesthesia. Thrombus from the common and superficial femoral artery was removed with an embolectomy catheter, restoring normal foot pulses after repair of the artery. Post-operatively, the patient was anti-coagulated with intravenous heparin and then warfarinised. She was discharged home 7 days later with an uneventful recovery.

Further reading

Berridge DC, Kessel DO, and Robertson I. Surgery versus thrombolysis for initial management of acute limb ischaemia. Cochrane Database of Systematic Reviews 2013, Issue 6. Art. No.: CD002784. DOI: 10.1002/14651858.CD002784.pub2.

Liapis CD and Kakisis JD. Acute ischaemia of the lower extremities. In: Liapis CD, Balzer K, Benedetti-Valentini F, and Fernandes e Fernandes J., eds. *European manual of medicine. Vascular surgery*. Springer-Verlag, Berlin, 2007, pp. 449–457.

Norgren L, Hiatt WR, Dormandy JA *et al.*, TASC II Working Group. Inter-society consensus for the management of peripheral arterial disease (TASC II). *J Vasc Surg* 2007;**45**(Suppl S):S5–S67.

O'Connell JB and Quiñones-Baldrich WJ. Proper evaluation and management of acute embolic versus thrombotic limb ischemia. *Semin Vasc Surg* 2009;**22**:10–16.

Wahlberg E, Olofsson P, and Goldstone J. Acute leg ischemia. In: *Emergency vascular surgery. A practical guide*. Springer-Verlag, Berlin, 2007, pp. 119–133.

CHAPTER 7

Chronic Lower Limb Ischaemia

Harjeet Rayt and Robert S.M. Davies

Department of Vascular and Endovascular Surgery, Leicester Royal Infirmary, UK

OVERVIEW

- Peripheral vascular disease (PVD) presents in many different ways ranging from intermittent claudication (IC) to critical limb ischaemia (CLI).
- Diagnosis of PVD indicates widespread atherosclerosis.
- Treatment of IC centres on risk factor modification and symptom relief.
- Treatment of CLI requires urgent referral to vascular services for limb revascularisation.
- Invasive treatment (angioplasty or bypass) is generally reserved for those with CLI, although severe lifestyle-limiting IC may be an indication.

Introduction

The phrase 'chronic lower limb ischaemia' refers to symptoms and signs of leg ischaemia that have been present for at least 2 weeks. This covers a wide range of disease from asymptomatic peripheral vascular disease (PVD) and intermittent claudication (IC) at one end of the spectrum to critical limb ischaemia (CLI) at the other (Table 7.1). For the purposes of this chapter, these extremes of disease will be considered individually. While the prevalence of symptomatic PVD in people aged 55–74 years is approximately 5%, 8% and 20% of this age group have asymptomatic major and minor disease, respectively. An important point to remember when assessing patients with chronic leg ischaemia is that the affected leg is part of a patient who must be assessed as a whole, both medically and socially.

Table 7.1 Fontaine classification of severity of peripheral arterial disease.

Stage	Symptoms	Description
I	Asymptomatic	PVD present but no symptoms
II	Intermittent claudication	Cramp-like pain in leg muscle on activity, eased with rest
III	Rest pain	Constant pain in feet (worse at night)
IV	Tissue loss	Ischaemic ulceration or gangrene

ABC of Arterial and Venous Disease, Third Edition.
Edited by Tim England and Akhtar Nasim.
© 2015 John Wiley & Sons, Ltd. Published 2015 by John Wiley & Sons, Ltd.

Definitions

Peripheral Arterial Disease (PAD)/Peripheral Vascular Disease (PVD). This is a vascular disease caused primarily by atherosclerosis and thromboembolic pathophysiological processes that alters the normal structure and function of the aorta, its visceral branches and the arteries of the lower extremity.

Intermittent Claudication. This is a clinical diagnosis given to the symptoms of painful muscle cramps, usually in the legs, that reliably occurs during exercise and is relieved by rest.

Critical Limb Ischaemia. This is defined as an history of more than 2 weeks of rest pain, ulcers or gangrene attributed to arterial steno-occlusive disease, with an ankle pressure of <50 mmHg or toe pressure <30 mmHg.

Risk factors for chronic ischaemia

The underlying pathophysiological process will predominately be atherosclerosis. Prevalence of arterial disease in the legs will be suggestive of disease in other arterial segments, in particular, coronary (40–60%) and cerebral (25–50%). The risk factors associated with PVD mirror those for ischaemic heart disease. Arterial disease is commonly seen after the age of 55, but in combination with other risk factors, it is increasingly seen at a younger age. Non-modifiable factors include age, race and gender. Modifiable risk factors include smoking, diabetes mellitus, hyperlipidaemia and hypertension.

Assessment

A large proportion of patients with PVD will remain undiagnosed due to either absent or atypical symptoms. The absence of symptoms may be due to the limitation of exercise from other causes (e.g. respiratory disease), mild disease and peripheral neuropathy. Of the symptomatic patients, one-third will present with IC. This is classically a debilitating muscular pain in the calf, thigh or buttock on exertion that occurs predictably at a fixed distance and is relieved by rest within 5 min of stopping. The muscular pain results from anaerobic muscle metabolism from an inadequate arterial supply. Atypical symptoms are common and are described as leg aches, tiredness or weakness; the patient may be able to walk through the pain, and the pain may not completely resolve with rest.

As the disease progresses, the claudication distance (distance at which the patient develops symptoms) declines, and the perfusion to the foot may become sufficiently compromised that the patient complains of 'rest pain'. This is pain in the foot in the absence of exercise and often initially occurs at night when the affected leg is in an elevated position and tissue perfusion pressure is lowered. The patient often describes being awoken by severe pain finding relief only upon placing the affected foot in a dependent position such that gravity aids tissue perfusion; some patients may only be pain free sleeping in a chair. If this persists for 2 weeks, the patient is said to have developed CLI, which can be confirmed by the aforementioned criteria.

Examination of the patient should address three important questions:

1 Is PAD present?
2 How severe is the disease and is the foot imminently threatened (CLI)?
3 What is the anatomical location of disease, e.g. aorta, femoral artery, multiple arterial segments?

The examination of any patient with suspected chronic lower limb ischaemia should comprise a complete cardiovascular assessment including blood pressure (BP) and pulse assessment in both arms, auscultation of the heart and carotid arteries and palpation of the abdomen for the presence of an abdominal aortic aneurysm.

The lower limbs should be carefully inspected; a common mistake is failure to examine in-between the toes or the heels for occult ulceration/tissue loss. In contrast to the acutely ischaemic limb, skin temperature may be an unreliable sign in CLI, but a unilaterally cold leg should alert the physician to the possibility of PAD. Capillary refill time and Buerger's test are also useful indicators of disease. A critically ischaemic foot may appear red and 'healthy' particularly in patients who have had their foot in dependence awaiting the consultation (Figure 7.1). This is known as a 'sunset' foot and occurs due to maximal skin capillary dilatation and is often mistaken for cellulitis by the unwary. However, on elevation of the foot, the severity of the ischaemia is revealed through skin pallor and venous guttering

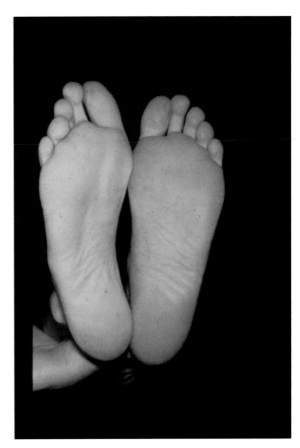

Figure 7.2 Photographic demonstration of elevation-induced pallor of the right leg indicating peripheral vascular disease. This is the basis of Buerger's test.

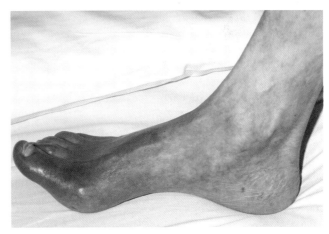

Figure 7.3 Photographic demonstration of a critically ischaemic foot with impending gangrene.

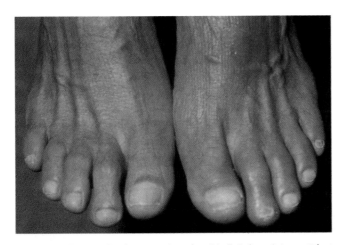

Figure 7.1 Photographic demonstration of a critically ischaemic 'sunset' foot (patient's left foot).

(Figure 7.2). Progression of the disease may lead to a blue/purple discolouration (Figure 7.3) before fixed changes such as gangrene become apparent (Figure 7.4).

Pulses throughout the lower limb should be assessed and documented. The muscle group affected by claudication is typically one anatomical level below the causative arterial stenosis/occlusion,

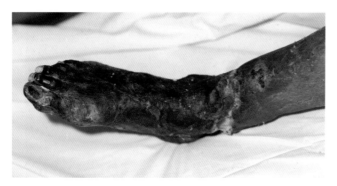

Figure 7.4 Photographic demonstration of dry gangrene.

i.e. the absence of palpable arterial pulses distal to the common femoral arterial denotes 'femoro-popliteal' arterial disease and may present as calf claudication, whereas weakness/absence of all lower limb arterial pulses including the common femoral pulse indicates aorto-iliac disease and often presents with calf, thigh and sometimes buttock symptomatology. It is important to remember that pedal pulses may be present at rest in patients with an isolated iliac system stenosis, but during exercise, the pulses may disappear as peripheral vasodilatation occurs.

Investigations

Hand-held Doppler examination gives vital information on the presence or absence of the peripheral pulses and should complete any vascular examination. Quantitative assessment can be made by performing an ankle brachial pressure index (ABPI) with a normal ratio being 0.9–1.3; ABPI values of 0.4–0.9 signify mild to moderate PAD, and values less than 0.4 are associated with severe PAD. Falsely elevated values (>1.3) may occur in patients with 'calcified' vessels (diabetics, chronic renal disease) and this should alert the clinician to the presence of PAD, although not necessarily flow-limiting PAD. The ABPI is usually performed at rest in the supine position. A simple advancement on baseline ABPI is to perform an ABPI after exercising to the onset of pain; the 'walk test'. A drop in the ABPI of ≥20% after exercise indicates the presence of flow-limiting PAD.

If vascular disease is suspected, the arterial tree can be imaged using duplex ultrasound scan (DUSS), or more complex investigations such as computed tomography arteriography (CTA), magnetic resonance arteriography (MRA) or percutaneous angiography (which can also be used as a therapeutic tool). DUSS is inexpensive, readily available and non-invasive, although it remains operator dependant. CTA is useful for assessing supra-inguinal arteries (aorto-iliac) that may be poorly visualised with DUSS due to vessel tortuosity, patient adiposity or overlying bowel gas. CTA is also readily available and can be used to create 3D reconstructions of the arterial tree, which aid in management planning. A major limitation in the use of CTA is the requirement for contrast media, which poses a risk of acute kidney injury (AKI) and allergic reaction. MRA also provides excellent imaging of the peripheral arterial tree with or without contrast (gadolinium). However, it is less readily available, contraindicated in patients with certain

types of metallic implants (pacemakers, stents) and not tolerated by claustrophobic patients. Digital subtraction angiography (percutaneous angiography) (DSA) is considered the 'gold standard' as it provides dynamic arterial flow information for the treating physician and can be combined with a definitive intervention in the form of angioplasty when indicated. However, it is invasive, expensive and associated with complications in ≤5% of patients that include AKI (from contrast use), allergic reaction, false aneurysm, arterial dissection, arteriovenous fistulation and embolisation.

Treatment

The overall aim of treating PVD is to (i) reduce the patient's cardiovascular risk through the modification/elimination of atherosclerotic risk factors and (ii) improve/relieve the patient's presenting symptomatology.

Risk factor modification

PVD is a strong marker of cardiovascular risk with over half of the patients having coronary artery disease; the extent of coronary artery disease has been shown to independently correlate with the patient's ABPI. Furthermore, more than one-quarter of patients with evidence of lower limb PVD have corresponding level of atherosclerotic disease affecting their carotid and renal arterial territories. Thus, it is not surprising that patients with PVD have a 6-fold increase in mortality from cardiovascular disease than their disease-free counterparts; *overall major cardiovascular event rate = 5–7% per year* (Figure 7.5).

Cardiovascular risk modification involves smoking cessation, diagnosis and control of diabetes mellitus and hypertension, diet and weight management, lipid modification and anti-platelet therapy. Smoking cessation can be achieved through a number of methods using formal cessation programmes and nicotine replacement therapy. The European Society of Cardiology recommends the maintenance of BP at ≤140/90 mmHg (with a systolic of ≤130 mmHg in diabetics and those with chronic kidney disease). Treatment with angiotensin-converting enzyme inhibitors (ACEi) is recommended as first line therapy due to benefits seen beyond simple BP control. Importantly, beta-blockers are

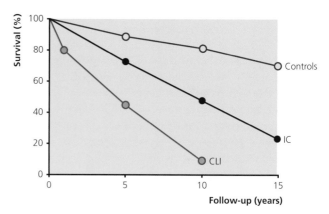

Figure 7.5 Survival in patients with IC and CLI compared with age-matched healthy controls. Source: Norgren *et al.* (2007). Reproduced by permission of Elsevier.

not contraindicated, and a recent meta-analysis found them not to affect claudication distance. HMG-CoA reductase inhibitors (statins) have been shown to reduce major cardiovascular events independent of age, gender or serum lipid levels. Anti-platelet agents have also shown a reduction in incidence of vascular mortality, and non-fatal MI/CVA of up to one-fifth.

'All patients with PVD should be commenced on anti-platelet therapy and a statin unless contraindicated and have appropriate measures instigated to control hypertension and diabetes'.

Symptom relief
Intermittent claudication
Asymptomatic disease does not require any treatment other than cardiovascular risk modification. Patients with IC should undergo a period of conservative management with the aim being symptom improvement by increasing claudication distance and reducing pain. This can be achieved through two main routes: exercise therapy and pharmacotherapy. Exercise not only improves symptoms but also works on multiple levels to reduce cardiovascular risk. NICE advises a formal programme that consists of 2 h of exercise a week for 3 months. The mechanism of action is unknown but theories regarding metabolic adaptation of muscle, change of muscle morphology and action, increased capillary blood flow and collateralisation have all been postulated. A number of studies have demonstrated that a structured exercise programme can lead to a sustained significant increase in peak walking distance without the need for invasive intervention.

Historically, a large number of drugs have been used to treat IC, but the evidence behind their use has been poor, and any benefits seen were minimal and short-lived. Currently, NICE recommends the use of naftidrofuryl oxalate only when exercise therapy has failed and the patient does not want invasive treatment. In the authors' experience, little 'real-life' benefit is gained through the use of pharmacotherapy for IC (Figure 7.6).

A number of patients will return to their treating doctor complaining that there has been little or no improvement in their presenting symptomatology. In these cases, particularly in those patients who are suffering from severe lifestyle-limiting claudication, invasive intervention in the form of angioplasty or bypass surgery may be considered. However, this must be discussed at length with the patient as resulting complications may lead to limb loss.

Critical limb ischaemia
Long-term survival of patients presenting with CLI is generally poor due to their advanced co-existent cardiovascular and cerebrovascular arterial disease. Twenty percent will die within a year and >50% die within 5 years. The aim of the treatment is 'life and limb' salvage (Figure 7.7).

Assessment in a vascular unit with a multidisciplinary approach is essential. Risk factor modification, wound care, footwear and rehabilitation can all be discussed before and after revascularisation. The mainstays of revascularisation are angioplasty and arterial bypass surgery. Choice of treatment depends on patient co-morbidities, pattern of disease, availability of a vein conduit and patient preference. Angioplasty is usually possible for iliac artery lesions up to 10 cm and superficial femoral artery (SFA) disease up to 15 cm (Figure 7.8). Longer lesions and crural disease can be attempted but require a greater level of skill. Bypass is generally performed using autologous long saphenous, cephalic or basilic vein grafts. In general, endovascular intervention is the preferred option for patients with significant co-morbidities, a life expectancy <2 years, grossly ulcerated/infected limbs rendering the integumentum unsuitable for surgical incisions and/or a lack of a suitable autologous vein conduit. Arterial bypass surgery is the preferred option in patients expected to survive beyond 2 years and is associated with 5-year limb salvage rates approaching 80% (Figure 7.9). In the authors' practice, a 'hybrid' approach is increasingly being employed where endovascular and open surgical revascularisation techniques are performed concomitantly.

Primary amputation may be considered in patients with extensive tissue loss, flexion contractures of the knee and hip and severe

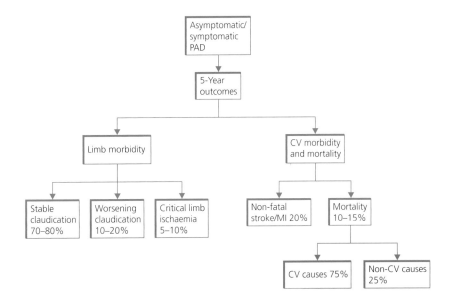

Figure 7.6 Intermittent claudication prognosis for patients and their legs.

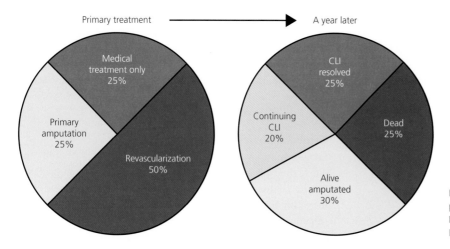

Primary treatment ⟶ A year later

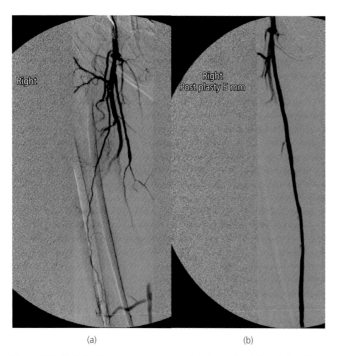

(a)   (b)

Figure 7.8 Digital subtraction angiogram showing before (a) and after (b) images of a long superficial femoral artery (SFA) angioplasty. Note the distal SFA on the left image supplied by collaterals.

Figure 7.7 Pie chart illustrating the fate of patients presenting with critical limb ischaemia. Source: Norgren *et al.* (2007). Reproduced by permission of Elsevier.

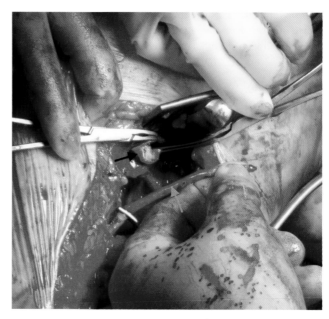

Figure 7.9 Intra-operative photograph before distal anastomosis of a femoropopliteal bypass graft. The blue arrow identifies the long saphenous vein conduit. The black arrow identifies the popliteal artery that has been opened with a longitudinal arteriotomy.

life-threatening sepsis. These decisions are best made involving the patient, relatives and the multidisciplinary team.

Occasionally, the option of revascularisation is not possible and the patient declines a major amputation. These patients are best placed on a formal palliative/end of life care pathway. NICE recommends using the analgesic ladder and recruiting the help of pain specialists; the majority of patients will require opioid analgesia for symptomatic relief. Chemical sympathectomy is not recommended by NICE.

Novel therapies

Spinal cord stimulation is a technique used for the relief of chronic pain. An epidural electrode is inserted and – using the pain gate theory – stimulation of the spinal cord at L3/4 has been shown to reduce pain and produce a sensation of warmth and paraesthesia in the limb. Results of this therapy are equivocal, and because of its high cost and side effects, it should only be offered by the pain team. Intermittent pneumatic compression has been shown to alleviate pain and healing by increasing blood flow, although the mechanism is not fully understood. While this remains a relatively cheap option, its effectiveness is yet to be proven. Iloprost, a synthetic analogue of prostacyclin PGI_2, has also been used to improve distal blood flow by causing a vasodilatory effect. However, it is usually administered intravenously, requiring hospital admission and can cause profound hypotension and headaches. Although studies have suggested a reduction in death and amputation with its use, these are not long-term effects. Angiogenesis and gene therapy are also being considered but these techniques at present remain research interests.

Clinical scenario: a patient with critical limb ischaemia

Presentation: A 67-year-old man was referred by his GP to the vascular clinic with a blackened left hallux and new onset rest pain, which developed in the previous 3–4 weeks. He was a life-long smoker and was on pharmacological treatment for hypertension and stable angina. He had a 6-month history of claudication but no history of diabetes mellitus.

Examination findings: Cold left foot with prolonged capillary refill and a 'dry' gangrenous hallux. A smaller area of ulceration was noted on the lateral malleolus. Absent left popliteal and ankle pulses. No motor or sensory dysfunction, no calf compression tenderness.

Diagnosis: CLI with tissue loss.

Investigations: Blood tests (FBC, U&Es, CRP, lipids & glucose), ABPI, arterial duplex scan.

Results: Blood tests were normal, ABPI decreased at 0.4, arterial duplex scan showed a short occlusion of left above knee popliteal artery.

Management: Anti-platelet therapy (aspirin 75 mg), statin therapy, risk factor modification and left leg SFA to below knee popliteal artery bypass. This patient most likely developed an acute thrombotic occlusion of a diseased popliteal artery with or without concomitant embolisation to the hallux causing tissue necrosis (gangrene).

Further reading

National Institute for Health and Clinical Excellence. Lower limb peripheral arterial disease: diagnosis and management (NICE clinical guideline 147), August 2012.

Norgren L, Hiatt WR, Dormandy JA *et al.*, TASC II Working Group. Inter-society consensus for the management of peripheral arterial disease (TASC II). *Eur J Vasc Endovasc Surg* 2007; **33**(Suppl.):S5-s67.

Slovut DP, Sullivan TM. Critical limb ischemia: medical and surgical management. *Vasc Med* 2008; **13**:281–291.

Tendra M, Aboyans V, *et al.* The Task force on the diagnosis and treatment of peripheral artery diseases of the European society of cardiology (ESC). ESC Guidelines on the diagnosis and treatment of peripheral artery diseases. *Eur Heart J* 2011;**32**:2851–1906.

CHAPTER 8

Venous Thromboembolic Disease

Harjeet Rayt and Akhtar Nasim

Department of Vascular & Endovascular Surgery, Leicester Royal Infirmary, UK

OVERVIEW

- Venous thromboembolism (VTE) is a common problem in hospitalised patients.
- Diagnosis of deep vein thrombosis (DVT) can be established by use of D-dimer testing and compression ultrasonography.
- Pulmonary embolism (PE) is a serious and often fatal complication of VTE.
- PE can be effectively diagnosed by computed tomography pulmonary angiography (CTPA).
- All at-risk patients must receive thromboprophylaxis.

Introduction

Venous thromboembolism (VTE) is the formation of a thrombus in a vein, which may dislodge from its original site and travel to a distant site (embolism). The commonest site for the formation of thrombus is the deep veins of the leg, hence the name deep vein thrombosis (DVT). The embolus may travel to the lungs and lodge in the pulmonary vasculature causing a pulmonary embolus (PE). It has been estimated that approximately 25 000 people in the United Kingdom die per annum from preventable hospital-acquired VTE. This has been highlighted by a recent UK study that suggested that 71% of the patients with medium or high risk of developing DVT did not receive any form of thromboprophylaxis. Non-fatal VTE is also important as it causes long-term morbidity such as post-phlebitic syndrome.

Deep vein thrombosis (DVT)

Typically, a DVT starts in the calf veins and presents with pain, swelling and erythema (Figure 8.1). Tenderness may be found in the thigh or calf, there may be unilateral pitting oedema and the patient may exhibit mild pyrexia. However, the symptoms of DVT can be vague and other differential diagnoses must also be considered (Box 8.1). The risk factors for DVT are listed in Table 8.1. Lower limb DVT can be subdivided into distal (calf) or proximal (thigh), with the greatest risk of PE arising from a proximal DVT.

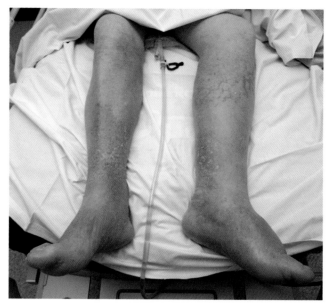

Figure 8.1 Photo of a patient with a left leg deep vein thrombosis.

Box 8.1 **Differential diagnosis of DVT**

- Calf muscle injury
- Acute lipodermatosclerosis
- Superficial thrombophlebitis
- Lymphatic insufficiency/lymphoedema
- Ruptured Baker's cyst
- Leg swelling in a paralysed limb
- Cellulitis
- Knee joint pathology
- Fracture
- Reperfusion injury/compartment syndrome

Pathophysiology

Rudolf Virchow (1821–1902) described a triad of factors that were broadly responsible for the formation of thrombosis. These are slowing in blood flow (stasis), changes in blood components (hypercoagulability) and damage to the vessel wall (venous injury). These factors are still responsible for DVT in modern practice. Stasis could be caused by immobility of the patient; hypercoagulability

ABC of Arterial and Venous Disease, Third Edition.
Edited by Tim England and Akhtar Nasim.
© 2015 John Wiley & Sons, Ltd. Published 2015 by John Wiley & Sons, Ltd.

Table 8.1 Risk factors for venous thromboembolism.

Acquired disorders	Inherited/congenital disorders
Malignancy	Antithrombin deficiency
Surgery, especially orthopaedic	Protein C deficiency
Presence of central venous catheter	Protein S deficiency
Trauma	Factor V Leiden mutation
Pregnancy, HRT, oral contraceptive	Prothrombin gene mutation
Prolonged immobilisation	Dysfibrinogenaemias
Dehydration	Factor VII deficiency
Age over 60	Factor XII deficiency
Obesity (BMI > 30)	
Previous VTE	
Congestive cardiac/respiratory failure	
Antiphospholipid syndrome	
Myeloproliferative disorders	
Poorly controlled diabetes mellitus	
Hyperviscosity syndromes (myeloma)	
Inflammatory bowel disease	
Acute medical illness	
Behcet's disease	
Varicose veins with associated phlebitis	

could be due to dehydration or effects of impaired coagulation and venous injury could be due to iatrogenic trauma or from the effects of inflammatory cytokines.

The thrombus usually forms close to the vein wall, usually in a valve pocket. This is rich in red blood cells and described as a red thrombus. As the thrombus propagates towards the lumen, more platelets and fibrin are involved and lead to a white appearance of the clot. From here, the clot either occludes the vein locally or forms a free-floating non-occlusive clot that can dislodge to a distant site.

Diagnosing DVT

Clinical diagnosis of DVT is unreliable and uses outdated historical tests such as Homan's sign. The most important serum investigation is a D-dimer test. The D-dimer examination has a high negative predictive value and can therefore be used to exclude a diagnosis of DVT if not elevated. However, an elevated value is non-specific and can occur in malignancy, pregnancy, recent surgery or trauma. Venography is the 'gold standard' diagnostic tool for DVT; however, its use is limited as the test can be painful and uses contrast medium (nephrotoxicity and anaphylaxis) (Figure 8.2). Venous ultrasonography is currently the investigation of choice. It is non-invasive, inexpensive, painless and readily accessible (Figure 8.3). It has a sensitivity and specificity of approximately 97% for the diagnosis of proximal DVT. A compression technique is used whereby the veins of a healthy vein can be opposed, whereas the walls of a vein containing thrombus remain apart (Figure 8.4). Computed tomography (CT), magnetic resonance imaging (MRI) and impedance plethysmography may also be used.

To avoid unnecessary investigation, several clinical prediction tools have been devised that incorporate symptoms, signs and risk factors to stratify patients into low or high risk for DVT (Table 8.2). This has been used along with D-dimer testing and ultrasonography to develop a diagnostic algorithm for patients with suspected DVT (Figure 8.5).

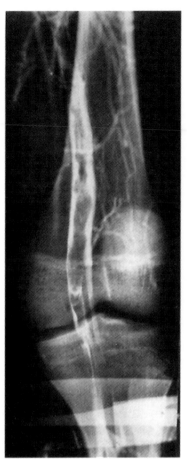

Figure 8.2 A venogram showing extensive thrombus (filling defect) in the popliteal vein.

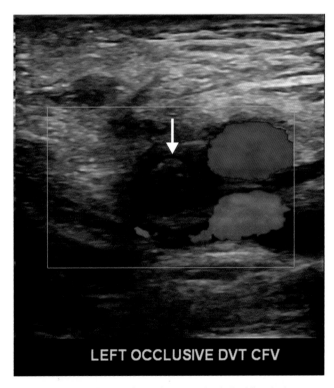

LEFT OCCLUSIVE DVT CFV

Figure 8.3 Duplex ultrasound scan demonstrating lack of flow in the common femoral vein indicating an occlusive DVT (arrow).

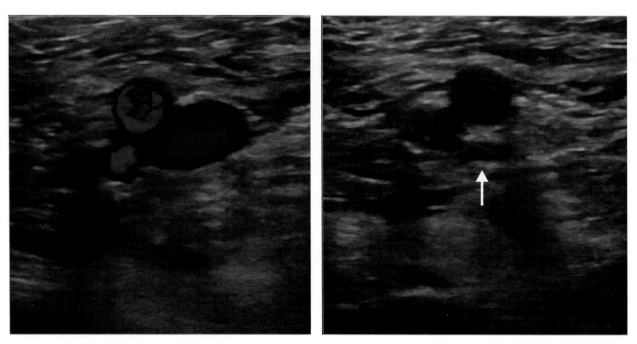

Figure 8.4 Normal duplex ultrasound scan demonstrating compression of the vein (arrow).

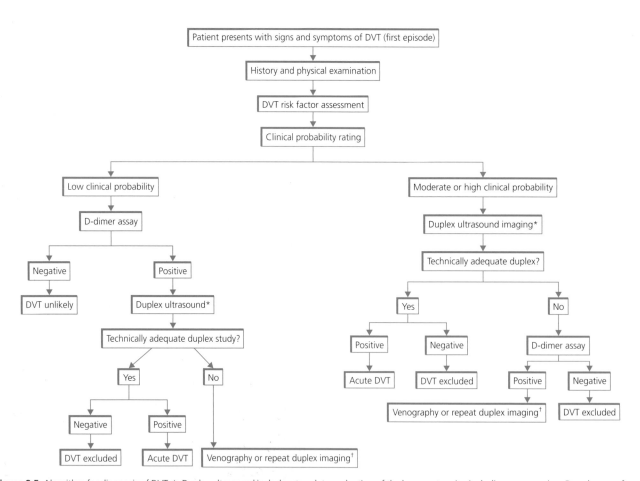

Figure 8.5 Algorithm for diagnosis of DVT. *, Duplex ultrasound includes complete evaluation of the lower extremity, including compression, Doppler waveforms, and colour Doppler of the calf veins and iliac veins. †, Contrast venography or magnetic resonance venography are warranted if the initial duplex study is technically inadequate or non-diagnostic. Source: Zierler (2004). Reproduced by permission of Wolters Kluwer Health.

Table 8.2 Clinical model for predicting pretest probability of DVT (Wells' score).

Clinical characteristics	Score
Active malignancy (ongoing treatment or palliative)	1
Immobilisation by paralysis or plaster dressings	1
Recently bedridden for >3 days or major surgery within previous 4 weeks	1
Localised tenderness along the distribution of the deep venous system	1
Whole leg swollen (thigh and calf)	1
Calf swelling >3 cm compared to asymptomatic leg (measured 10 cm below tibial tuberosity)	1
Pitting oedema (confined to symptomatic leg)	1
Collateral superficial veins (non-varicosed)	1
Previous documented DVT	1
Alternative diagnosis at least as likely as DVT	−2

Source: Zierler (2004). Reproduced by permission of Wolters Kluwer Health.
DVT likely if score ≥2, unlikely if score ≤1.
Low probability of DVT 0; high probability ≥3.

Complications of DVT

The main complications of DVT are pulmonary embolism (PE), venous insufficiency and recurrent thrombosis.

Pulmonary embolism

PE is a serious complication of DVT, with a reported 30-day mortality rate of approximately 10%. A massive PE results from a large embolus that obstructs the main pulmonary artery, leads to acute right ventricular failure and can be fatal. Smaller emboli lodge more distally in the pulmonary arterial tree and cause cardiorespiratory symptoms (Box 8.2). Diagnosing PE always requires a high index of suspicion as some may present with very little symptoms. Most PE are multiple and commonly affect the lower lobes. The 'gold standard' for diagnosis is a pulmonary angiogram. This is an expensive, invasive test that requires trained radiologists and co-operative patients and has therefore largely been reserved for patients in whom non-invasive tests are inconclusive. Computed tomography pulmonary angiography (CTPA) has now taken over as the investigation of choice for diagnosing PE. This is a non-invasive, fast, widely available test that allows visualisation of the entire lung fields as well as the pulmonary tree (Figure 8.6). Alternative diagnoses can therefore be determined. However, problems with the above-mentioned investigations are high radiation exposures, which can be problematic in pregnancy and contrast media and may cause nephrotoxicity or anaphylaxis. In these circumstances, a ventilation/perfusion scan is a safer alternative. Treatment for PE centres around anticoagulation and supportive cardiorespiratory measures. Massive PE resulting in haemodynamic compromise (hypoxia, tachycardia and hypotension) is an indication for thrombolysis. Surgical management of massive PE is no longer recommended.

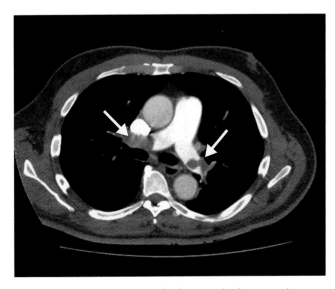

Figure 8.6 CT pulmonary angiography demonstrating large extensive bilateral pulmonary emboli (arrows).

Post-thrombotic venous insufficiency

DVT can lead to venous valve damage, resulting in valvular incompetence. A combination of deep vein reflux and venous obstruction from unresolved thrombus leads to post-thrombotic venous insufficiency (also known as post-phlebitic syndrome). The cumulative incidence of this condition is 17, 23 and 28% at 1, 2 and 5 years, respectively, with no increase thereafter. It results in lower leg swelling, pain, skin pigmentation and venous ulcers (Figure 8.7). The trophic skin changes (haemosiderin deposition, lipodermatosclerosis, atrophie blanche and skin ulceration) tend to occur 2–4 years after a DVT. The use of class II compression hosiery in patients with DVT has been shown to reduce the incidence of this complication.

Recurrent thrombosis

The recurrence of DVT is associated with a high risk of further thromboembolic events. Therefore, such patients should probably continue with life-long anticoagulation.

Treatment of DVT

Aims of treatment of VTE are symptom relief, prevention of thrombus propagation and prevention of recurrent thrombosis.

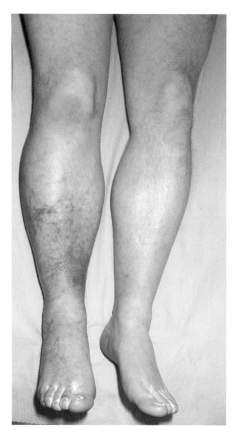

Figure 8.7 A photograph showing the typical skin changes observed in patients with post-thrombotic venous insufficiency (right leg).

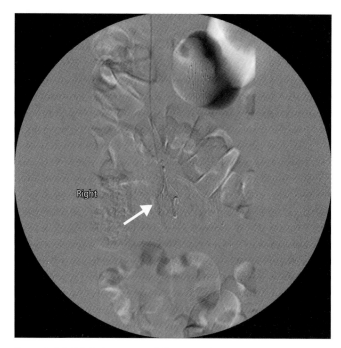

Figure 8.8 IVC (inferior vena cava) filter *in situ* (arrow). Also note the presence of an endovascular AAA (abdominal aortic aneurysms) device.

Anticoagulation

This should be commenced once the diagnosis is suspected and a risk assessment is favourable. Treatment should not be delayed for confirmation of the diagnosis by investigations. Anticoagulation aims to prevent the propagation of thrombus and PE in the short term and prevent recurrent events in the long term. Anticoagulation is further discussed in Chapter 15.

Inferior vena cava filter

These act as a physical barrier for the prevention of emboli and hence reduce the rate of PE (Figure 8.8). They are indicated in patients who cannot be safely anticoagulated (recent haemorrhage, impending surgery) or patients who continue to develop PE despite adequate anticoagulation (Chapter 15).

Thrombolysis

More recently, apart from the treatment of massive PE, thrombolysis has been used in the treatment of DVT. This can be given locally via an endoluminal catheter to minimise the systemic side effects and is used to prevent the development of post-phlebitic syndrome. However, the evidence for this remains unclear. Another use is in patients with large ileofemoral DVT with impending limb gangrene despite adequate anticoagulation.

Prevention of VTE disease

All patients should be assessed on admission to identify their risk for developing VTE.

Mechanical

Thromboembolism deterrent stockings (TEDS) reduce venous stasis in the lower leg by applying a graded degree of compression from the ankle to the calf, with greater pressure being applied distally. They are simple and safe to use but are contraindicated in patients with arterial insufficiency or diabetic neuropathy. Below knee elastic compression hosiery (class II) work in a similar way but can reduce oedema and prevent skin blistering from venous hypertension. Use of these stockings following a DVT reduces the risk of developing post-phlebitic venous insufficiency. Intra-operatively, intermittent pneumatic compression wraps may be applied.

Pharmacological

In addition to the above-mentioned mechanical prophylaxis, patients at increased risk of VTE (at least one risk factor from Table 8.1) should be commenced on low molecular weight heparin (LMWH). This is preferred to unfractionated heparin due to its enhanced bioavailability, side effect profile (reduced incidence of heparin-induced thrombocytopenia) and dosage regime. Fondaparinux may be used as an alternative to LMWH and has been shown to be more effective than LMWH in preventing VTE in orthopaedic surgery. Its limitations arise from its cost and longer half-life.

Current NICE guidelines (clinical guideline 92) recommend that patients undergoing non-orthopaedic surgery should have mechanical prophylaxis at admission if not contraindicated and be commenced on pharmacological prophylaxis (if bleeding risk is low) up to a period of time when mobility is no longer reduced. A choice of LMWH, fondaparinux or unfractionated heparin is suggested. In elective orthopaedic surgery, a similar approach is taken, but pharmacological treatments are continued for a minimum of 10 days, with dabigatran and rivroxaban added to the list of recommended anticoagulants. Different regimes are suggested for emergency orthopaedic surgery. The VTE thromboprophylaxis regime should be reviewed regularly on ward rounds, especially after clinical interventions.

Clinical scenario: a patient with deep vein thrombosis

Presentation: A 72-year-old woman presents to accident and emergency with a swollen left leg over the past week. She is currently undergoing chemotherapy for recently diagnosed breast cancer and wonders whether it is a side effect of the treatment. She is a current smoker and treated for hypertension.

Examination: Generally, she appears well. She is in sinus rhythm and her abdominal examination is unremarkable. Her left leg is markedly more swollen than the right with pitting oedema in the lower leg. There is some mild tenderness in the calf. She has a palpable femoral and popliteal pulse and although the foot is warm, no foot pulses are palpable, possibly due to the oedema.

Differential diagnoses: DVT, ruptured Baker's cyst and lymphoedema.

Investigations: Blood tests (including D-dimer) and venous duplex.

Results: Elevated D-dimer with mild thrombocytosis and venous duplex shows large ileofemoral DVT.

Management: Anticoagulation (therapeutic LMWH, then warfarin), analgesia, compression hosiery and limb elevation.

Outcome: Leg swelling and pain gradually reduced. Patient was warfarinised successfully with a view to re-assessing this in 6 months.

Further reading

Department of Health and Chief Medical Officer. Report of the independent expert working group on the prevention of venous thromboembolism in hospitalised patients, 2007. Available from http://www.dh.gov.uk/prod_consum_dh/groups/dh_digitalassets/documents/digitalasset/dh_073950.pdf.

National Clinical Guidance Centre. Venous thromboembolic diseases: the management of venous thromboembolic diseases and the role of thrombophilia testing. Clinical Guideline. Methods, evidence and recommendations, June 2012.

National Institute for Health and Clinical Excellence. Venous thromboembolism: reducing the risk. Reducing the risk of venous thromboembolism (deep vein thrombosis and pulmonary embolism) in patients admitted to hospital. NICE clinical guideline 92, January 2010.

Zierler BK. Ultrasonography and diagnosis of venous thromboembolism. *Circulation* 2004;**109**:I-9–I-14.

CHAPTER 9

Varicose Veins

Greg S. McMahon and Mark J. McCarthy

Department of Vascular & Endovascular Surgery, Leicester Royal Infirmary, UK

> ## OVERVIEW
>
> - Varicose veins are common, affecting around one-third of the adult population in the developed world.
> - The clinical presentation of varicose veins is variable, from cosmetic issues to severe limb-threatening ulceration.
> - Most patients with uncomplicated varicose veins will never progress to develop skin changes or ulceration, and can be appropriately reassured.
> - NICE (National Institute for Health and Care Excellence) guidance recommends that for complicated varicose veins, endovenous ablation should be the first-line treatment, followed by foam sclerotherapy, then surgery.
> - All patients with skin changes and those undergoing intervention should be assessed with colour Doppler ultrasonography primarily.

Introduction

Varicose veins are common. While estimates vary, prevalence is probably in the region of a quarter to one-third of the adult population, and in 2009, over 30 000 varicose vein procedures were carried out on the National Health Service (NHS). The word 'varicose' describes (often tortuous) dilatation of a vein, a process that, while theoretically affecting any vein in the body, is most commonly encountered in the leg, due to the hydrostatic pressure of upright positioning (Figure 9.1). The symptoms of varicose veins are wide-ranging, from none through to mild cosmetic issues, to very severe symptoms including ulceration.

Pathophysiology

Varicose veins are almost always the result of superficial venous reflux or incompetence (i.e. flow retrograde to the physiological norm), which is usually due to failure of the venous valve mechanism. Valve failure is either *primary* – a dysfunction of the leaflets or annulus itself – or *secondary* – a weakness in the vein wall that results in widening of the valve leaflets, and ensuing incompetence

due to their incomplete apposition. While it is likely that varicose veins result from a combination of these mechanisms, there is evidence to suggest that patients with varicose veins do indeed have an inherent reduction in vein wall elasticity. This would, in part, explain why recurrence of varicose veins is so common following treatment (5%). Furthermore, it is proposed that there is a hereditary component to varicose veins; the observation that the children of two parents with varicose veins have a 90% chance of developing them is compelling.

There are other risk factors for the development of varicose veins including female sex, prolonged standing, increased height, obesity (through venous hypertension), increasing age and multiparity. More rarely, varicose veins are the result of deep vein thrombosis, pelvic tumour or vascular malformation.

Classification

The distinction between 'thread' or 'spider' veins and other varicosities is simply based on size, with the former referring to intra-dermal venules of less than 1-mm diameter (Figure 9.1). Valvular dysfunction can be present in the long (or greater) saphenous or short (or lesser) saphenous veins, or their major tributaries in which case the term 'trunk' or 'truncal' varicosity is used. Valvular incompetence does not need to be present in one of the trunk veins for large varicosities to occur; where varicose veins develop because of local dysfunction in an unnamed tributary, the veins are sometimes termed 'reticular'.

The CEAP (clinical, aetiological, anatomical, and pathophysiological) classification (Table 9.1) is now the worldwide standard for describing in detail the clinical features of chronic venous disease. This thorough tool has probably found its niche more as a common language for the comparison of research trials rather than as a widespread clinical aid in daily practice.

Clinical presentation

Varicose veins are often cited as responsible for a variety of symptoms, including sensations of heaviness, burning, cramping, itching, tingling and aching. Such symptoms could equally be attributed to other vascular and non-vascular conditions and it is sometimes difficult to prove a cause-and-effect relationship between varicose veins and a patient's symptoms. The authors of the Edinburgh Vein

---

ABC of Arterial and Venous Disease, Third Edition.
Edited by Tim England and Akhtar Nasim.
© 2015 John Wiley & Sons, Ltd. Published 2015 by John Wiley & Sons, Ltd.

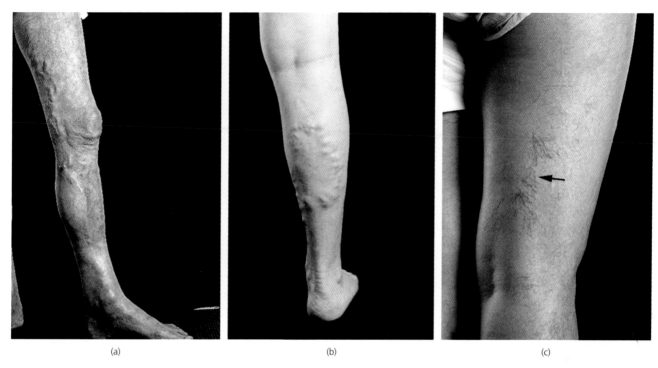

(a) (b) (c)

Figure 9.1 Trunal varices are varicosities in the line of the long (a) or short (b) saphenous vein or their major branches. Reticular veins (c) are dilated tortuous subcutaneous veins not belonging to the main branches of the long or short saphenous vein and telangiectasia (c) are intra-dermal venules less than 1 mm in size. (c) Demonstrates both reticular veins and telangiectasia. The latter are also referred to as 'spider veins', 'star bursts', 'thread veins' or 'matted veins'.

Table 9.1 CEAP (clinical, aetiological, anatomical, and pathophysiological) classification of severity and aetiology of lower limb venous disease.

Clinical classification		Aetiological classification		Anatomical classification		Pathophysiological classification	
C0	No signs of venous disease	Ec	Congenital	As	Superficial veins	Pr	Reflux
C1	Reticular veins	Ep	Primary	Ap	Perforator veins	Po	Obstruction
C2	Varicose veins	Es	Secondary (post-thrombotic)	Ad	Deep veins	Pr,o	Reflux and obstruction
C3	Oedema	En	No venous cause identified	An	No venous location identified	Pn	No venous pathophysiology identified
C4a	Pigmentation or eczema						
C4b	Lipodermatosclerosis or atrophie blanche						
C5	Healed venous ulcer						
C6	Active venous ulcer						
S	Symptomatic						
A	Asymptomatic						

Study investigated this uncertainty and concluded that even in the presence of trunk varicosities, most lower limb symptoms probably do not have a venous cause. It is in the management of patient expectation that this finding has its important implication.

There is no doubt, however, that varicose veins can be responsible for significant changes in the skin of the lower leg, and this is usually best demonstrated at the ankle. The skin changes are thought to be the result of abnormal pressures within the venous system induced by the reflux, and subsequent extravasation of blood into the tissues. They range from pigmentation caused by the deposition in the skin

of haemosiderin (Figure 9.2), eczema (Figure 9.3), atrophie blanche (Figure 9.4) and lipodermatosclerosis (Figure 9.5) to overt ulceration (Figure 9.6). Again, when considering patient concerns, it is worthwhile acknowledging that ulceration is actually relatively rare.

While the skin changes are due to abnormalities in venous haemodynamics, other complications of varicose veins are related to the veins themselves. For example, when bleeding occurs, it is most commonly from varicosities at the ankle and can be profuse. Thrombophlebitis is inflammation of the vein wall secondary to thrombosis and is commonly a recurrent phenomenon (Figure 9.7).

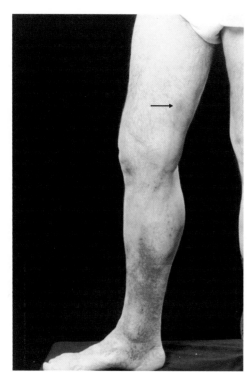

Figure 9.2 Skin pigmentation is due to haemosiderin deposition and is most commonly situated above the medial malleolus. However, it may encircle the entire ankle and extend up the leg. In addition, this patient has thrombophlebitis of the long saphenous vein with overlying pigmentation (arrow).

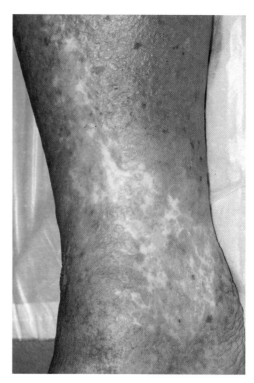

Figure 9.4 Atrophie blanche results from skin necrosis followed by scarring. Sometimes, small areas of atrophie blanche coalesce to form a large scar.

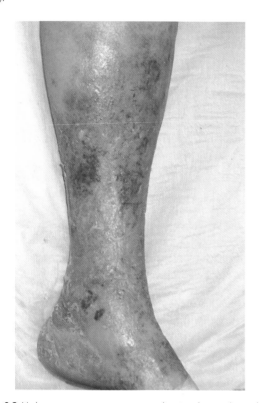

Figure 9.3 Varicose eczema occurs over prominent varicose veins and in the lower third of the leg. It may be dry, scaly and vesicular or 'weeping and ulcerated'. A generalised sensitisation may occur leading to patches elsewhere.

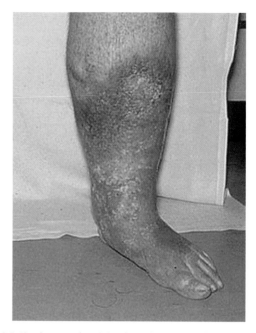

Figure 9.5 Lipodermatosclerosis involving the medial calf. Acute lipodermatosclerosis presents with a painful, tender, hot, raised red-brown area on the lower leg. The chronic form leads to a hard, indurated area on the lower leg with a palpable edge. The overlying skin is often brown and shiny. The progressive contraction of the gaiter area gives the leg an 'inverted champagne bottle' appearance.

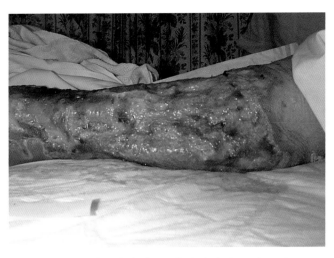

Figure 9.6 Venous ulcer, classically seen in the 'gaiter' area; lower leg, medial aspect, frequently in an area of skin displaying other evidence of venous incompetence.

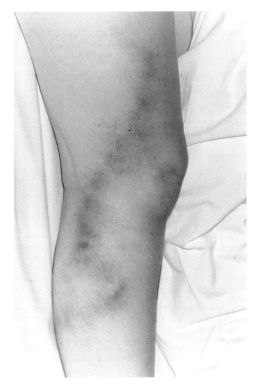

Figure 9.7 Thrombophlebitis caused by a reaction to superficial venous thrombosis. If this approaches the saphenofemoral vein junction, the patient is at risk of deep venous thrombosis and pulmonary embolism.

Patient assessment

History

Why is the patient seeking treatment? Do they have symptoms attributable to varicose veins? Is there an alternative explanation for their leg symptoms? Do they have evidence of arterial, musculoskeletal or neurological pathology, for example? Management of the patient's concerns and expectations is paramount. It is important also to determine any known history of deep vein

thrombosis, or of any conditions that would increase the risk of venous thrombotic events (pregnancies, leg fractures, thrombophilias). This not only helps in distinguishing the aetiology of the presenting complaint, it also has an impact on management decisions; a history of deep vein thrombosis or thrombophlebitis increases the risk of peri-procedural thrombosis should there be intervention.

Examination

Examination has three objectives: to look for a possible cause of the venous insufficiency, to examine the status of the peripheral arterial system, and to examine the varicose veins themselves. An abdominal examination should be performed to look for any masses that could be causing venous obstruction, and an arterial examination should be undertaken to determine the contribution of peripheral vascular disease to the patient's symptoms and to rule out significant arterial insufficiency that may complicate future management options.

Examination of varicose veins is best performed in a warm room, with the patient standing. In addition to assessing the distribution of the varicosities, scars from previous varicose vein interventions can be looked for. With the evolution of more modern adjuncts, tourniquet tests are generally considered unreliable and are certainly insufficient for the planning of intervention. Although hand-held continuous wave Doppler can reliably identify the site of incompetence in the majority of cases of varicose veins, it is limited in patients with recurrent varicose veins and in instances where there is more than one site of incompetence. Furthermore, it provides no information about the deep venous system.

Investigation

While for many years considered mandatory for patients with skin changes, recurrent varicose veins or deep vein thrombosis, evidence increasingly suggests that colour duplex ultrasonography should actually be carried out on all patients for whom varicose vein intervention is to be considered. It is affordable, non-invasive and relatively simple to perform and is the only method capable of assessing the deep system, as well as giving accurate information on the exact anatomy of the venous incompetence. The most recent guidance issued from the National Institute for Health and Care Excellence (NICE) recommends that ultrasound be used routinely in this setting.

Treatment

While evidently a concern, most patients with uncomplicated varicose veins will actually never progress to develop skin changes, ulceration or deep vein thrombosis and they can be confidently reassured that no intervention is necessary. NICE advises that patients should be referred to a vascular service if they have symptomatic varicose veins, skin changes, thrombophlebitis or a history of venous ulceration. For those in whom truncal reflux is confirmed, endothermal ablation with phlebectomies should be offered as a first-line treatment, provided the patient (and their venous anatomy) is suitable.

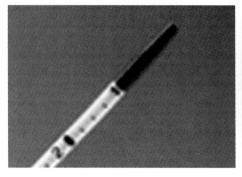

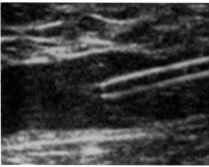

Figure 9.8 EVLT (endovenous laser treatment) catheter tip. The duplex image shows the catheter within the long saphenous vein.

Radiofrequency and endovenous laser ablation techniques are similar in that both deliver energy directly to the lumen of the vein via an intravenous catheter placed percutaneously under ultrasound guidance (Figure 9.8). The energy causes destruction of the vein wall with the aim of generating fibrotic occlusion of the refluxing trunk and its consequent exclusion from the venous system. The advantages of these techniques are that they are performed under local rather than general anaesthetic, as day-case procedures. They are particularly attractive for recurrent varicose veins as they avoid the necessity for difficult redo groin dissection. Adverse tortuosity of the superficial veins is a relative contraindication as this tends to preclude satisfactory passage of the ablating catheter. Where veins lie particularly superficially, the overlying skin is at risk of thermal injury – a judgement must be made as to whether ablation is safe.

If the patient is not suitable for endothermal ablation, ultrasound-guided foam sclerotherapy should be offered. This technique is also performed on a day-case basis without general anaesthesia and, like the ablation techniques, does not mandate the utilisation of a formal operating theatre environment. Sclerotherapy involves infusion of a foamed sclerosant into a collapsed vein with the effect of causing apposition long enough for occlusive fibrosis to occur; however, it can lead to skin pigmentation (Figure 9.9). The advantage of using a foamed sclerosant is that it effectively displaces the blood from the vessel and can be easily seen with ultrasound.

NICE guidance recommends that surgery be reserved for those individuals for whom the less invasive techniques are unsuitable. Surgery aims to treat the source of the venous incompetence, whether this is at the saphenofemoral vein junction, saphenopopliteal vein junction, at a perforator or through a recurrence. While open surgery can usually be performed as a day-case, it almost always necessitates a general anaesthetic and a formal theatre facility.

Compression hosiery may have a place in the management of varicose veins but in fact evidence for its benefit is weak. Therapy may relieve symptoms and prevent progression of skin changes, but stockings tend to be poorly tolerated (and subsequently irregularly applied) and they have to be worn indefinitely. As a result, NICE recommends that compression hosiery be reserved for those patients in whom other intervention is unsuitable.

Each of the invasive options carries the risk of recurrence and also of deep vein thrombosis, the latent incidence of which is probably slightly higher than the very small clinically manifest rate. In an attempt to reduce the thromboembolic risk of intervention, many surgeons administer heparin or low molecular weight heparin peri-operatively and some also advise patients taking hormone supplements to cease these around the time of treatment.

There remains a relative paucity of randomised and long-term outcome data for the non-surgical procedures but there is mounting evidence to support the assertion that their efficacy is likely to be at least similar to that of the traditional open surgical techniques.

Treatment of complications

Thrombophlebitis is a sterile inflammation, and, therefore, there is no indication for treatment with antibiotics. Instead, treatment consists of anti-inflammatories (systemic or topical) and analgesia. While compression is theoretically useful to reduce thrombus propagation, the reality is that this is often intolerable for an already painful leg. Referral to a vascular specialist is warranted, as intervention is frequently required for the abnormal vein in order to prevent recurrent episodes of inflammation. It is of particular concern when the thrombophlebitis tracks along the long saphenous vein in the thigh, as there is a risk of propagation of the thrombus across the saphenofemoral vein junction and into the deep system. This can usually be determined with duplex ultrasonography and should be treated with formal anticoagulation just as for a deep vein thrombosis. In addition, some surgeons advocate urgent operative disconnection and ligation of the saphenofemoral vein junction with extraction of the propagating thrombus under temporary deep venous control.

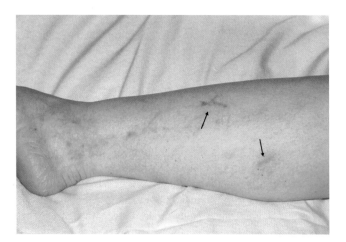

Figure 9.9 One of the complications of injection sclerotherapy is brown skin pigmentation (arrows).

Haemorrhage from varicose veins is alarming for the patient and can on occasion be significant. It is usually easily remediable acutely with elevation of the leg and direct pressure on the bleeding point. A vascular surgeon should see the patient, with a view to treating the underlying venous abnormality.

Patients with ulceration or skin changes should undergo colour duplex ultrasound assessment to define the venous abnormality. Pure superficial reflux should generally be treated, but in the presence of deep venous incompetence, ablating the superficial veins will not improve the skin. In this situation, the mainstay of treatment is compression therapy.

Clinical scenario: a patient with symptomatic varicose veins

Presentation: A 48-year-old female was referred to vascular surgery out-patients with troublesome right leg varicose veins. The varicose veins were longstanding but 6 months before being referred she developed a lower leg ulcer. This slowly healed but she then developed significant pain and tenderness in the calf varicosities. She had a background of HOCM (hypertrophic obstructive cardiomyopathy) and implantable defibrillator.

Examination findings: Long saphenous territory varicose veins with mildly tender and swollen (non-compressible) calf varicosities with associated skin inflammation. Skin changes in the lateral malleolar area consistent with haemosiderosis, varicose eczema and a healed ulcer. Full complement of arterial pulses. CEAP classification 5.

Differential diagnosis: superficial venous reflux, post-thrombotic venous insufficiency and stasis dermatitis.

Investigations: Venous duplex scan at the time of clinic attendance.

Results: Venous duplex demonstrated long saphenous reflux and evidence of partially occlusive thrombus in the calf varicosities consistent with resolving phlebitis.

Management: Prescribed non-steroidal anti-inflammatory (ibuprofen) and class II compression hosiery to treat the thrombophlebitis. Subsequently underwent successful endovenous laser ablation of long saphenous reflux under local anaesthetic to prevent recurrent phlebitis and skin ulceration.

Further reading

Bradbury A, Evans C, Allan P, *et al*. What are the symptoms of varicose veins? Edinburgh vein study cross sectional population survey. *BMJ*, 1999;**318**:353–356.

Eklöf B, Rutherford J, Bergan JJ *et al*. on behalf of the American venous forum international ad hoc committee for revision of the CEAP classification. *J Vasc Surg*, 2004;**40**:1248–1252.

Hamdan A. Management of varicose veins and venous insufficiency. *JAMA*, 2012;**24**:2612-2621.

National Institute for Health and Clinical Excellence (NICE). Varicose veins in the legs: the diagnosis and management of varicose veins: clinical guideline CG168. guidance.nice.org.uk/cg168. Issued July 2013.

CHAPTER 10

Lower Limb Ulceration

Huw O.B. Davies and J. Mark Scriven

Heart of England NHS FT, Birmingham, UK

OVERVIEW

- Lower limb ulceration affects around 3% of the elderly population.
- Has significant impact on the patient's quality of life and also places a large financial burden on the NHS.
- Common causes include varicose veins/venous disease, arterial disease and diabetes mellitus.
- Once the correct diagnosis has been made, most leg ulcers can be managed in the primary care setting.
- Atypical appearance or a non-healing ulcer should raise suspicion of skin malignancy and requires ulcer biopsy and histopathology.
- Venous ulcers can be healed successfully with compression bandaging applied in the community. However, associated superficial venous reflux may require treatment to prevent ulcer recurrence.

Introduction

One percent of the general population suffers from lower limb ulceration and this prevalence increases with age (3% of over 65-year-olds are affected). The management of leg ulcers often involves frequent visits to care providers (community nurses, tissue viability specialists, podiatrists, secondary care nurses, general practitioners, diabetologists, dermatologists, plastic surgeons and vascular surgeons) and non-healing ulceration increases the risk of lower limb amputation. Thus, chronic persistence and frequent ulcer recurrence places a large financial burden upon the NHS (estimated at £400–600 million annually). There is also a significant effect on patients' quality of life: ulcers can be painful, malodorous and may necessitate prolonged bandage treatment. As a result, patients can feel stigmatised and become socially isolated.

Table 10.1 details the causes of leg ulceration, the most common of which is vascular insufficiency. Venous ulceration accounts for over 75% of cases, the remaining aetiologies comprising arterial disease (2%), arteriovenous disease (12%) and the remaining due to other pathologies as described later. As the aetiology of lower limb ulceration spans a range of pathologies and thus will present in varying guises to primary care, such a structured, evidence-based approach to management is imperative. However, once an initial assessment and diagnosis has been made, most leg ulcers can subsequently be managed in a primary care setting.

Lower limb ulceration clinical assessment

Assessment of the underlying cause of ulceration is the key to ongoing management; this will direct treatment of both the primary ulcer and the underlying pathology. Box 10.1 outlines a pragmatic management pathway for patients presenting with lower limb ulceration. This combined with clinical assessment allows appropriate investigation and referral to specialist care.

Clinical history

Assessment of a patient's ulcer begins with a thorough history. Location, size, duration, pain and recurrence will guide the clinician towards a diagnosis. Co-morbid conditions should also be enquired about – diabetes, peripheral vascular disease, autoimmune disease, inflammatory bowel disease and connective tissue disorders as well as medication should be recorded. Previous arterial or venous interventions may give a clue to aetiology. Although eliciting a history of varicose veins is important, it is worth remembering that a proportion of patients with significant venous reflux have no varicosities apparent on clinical examination.

Social factors may also contribute to lower limb ulceration. Smoking is a known cause of peripheral vascular disease. Occupation may also contribute – particularly those who stand for long periods of the working day. Elderly people with decreased mobility possibly to the extent of spending most of the day sitting in a chair with oedematous dependent legs will have reduced calf muscle pump function and be at risk of ulceration. Muscle pump stasis also occurs as a result of morbid obesity that has a bearing when treatment options are considered.

Poorly controlled diabetes not only causes neuropathy but also an increased prevalence of lower limb infection and poor wound healing.

ABC of Arterial and Venous Disease, Third Edition.
Edited by Tim England and Akhtar Nasim.
© 2015 John Wiley & Sons, Ltd. Published 2015 by John Wiley & Sons, Ltd.

Table 10.1 Causes of lower limb ulceration.

"Vascular"
- Venous disease
- Arterial disease
- Mixed arteriovenous disease
- Vasculitis
- Severe hypertension (Martorell's ulcer)

Neuropathy
- Diabetic ulcers

Trauma/factitious

Malignancy
- Basal cell carcinoma
- Squamous carcinoma
- Melanoma
- Lymphoma (T cell mycosis fungoides, B cell)
- Sarcoma

Underlying osteomyelitis

Immobility/obesity

Lymphoedema

Steroid medication

Blood dyscrasias
- Sickle cell disease
- Thalassaemia
- Thrombotic thrombocythaemia

Skin conditions
- Necrobiosis lipoidica diabeticorum
- Pyoderma gangrenosum

Infection
- Cellulitis
- Yaws (*Treponema pertenue*)
- Syphilis
- Cutaneous anthrax
- Cutaneous tuberculosis
- Leprosy
- Parasites

Nutritional deficiency
- Vitamin C
- Zinc

Physical examination

Evaluation of the venous and arterial systems will commonly yield a cause for ulceration. It is therefore important to examine both of these systems thoroughly followed by a detailed assessment of the skin and ulcer. Absence of arterial or venous signs may indicate a rarer cause for ulceration and careful consideration regarding biopsy should be made.

Venous assessment

Evaluate both limbs for signs of chronic venous insufficiency (CVI). These include prominent varicose or reticular veins, brawny skin and venous eczema. Haemosiderin deposition and lipodermatosclerosis should also be noted.

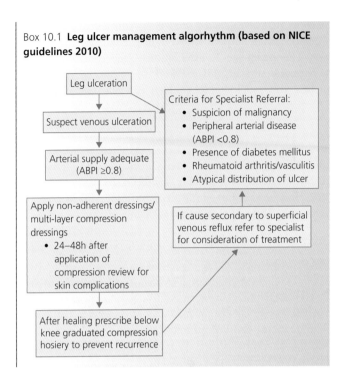

Box 10.1 **Leg ulcer management algorhythm (based on NICE guidelines 2010)**

Arterial assessment

Again both limbs should be assessed for the presence or absence of palpable lower limb pulses. Trophic changes associated with chronic arterial insufficiency may be present (pale, shiny skin that is often hairless).

The ankle-brachial pressure index (ABPI) should be measured to assess the degree of any underlying arterial pathology. Care should be taken in interpretation of results in diabetics who may have falsely elevated readings due to vessel calcification. An ABPI > 0.8 excludes a significant ischaemic component and would permit the safe use of compression bandages or hosiery if required to treat venous hypertension. If arterial disease is significant, then further imaging with a view to revascularisation would be indicated.

Ulcer assessment

Location is particularly helpful to determining the underlying cause but bear in mind that an atypical presentation of common ulcers does occur. Size should also be noted (it may be helpful to use serial measurement to assess response to treatment) and the ulcer's shape and sides should be noted along with the appearance of the base. The clinician should assess for superimposed infection (possibly requiring treatment with antibiotics or debridement) by examining surrounding skin also, compression of surrounding tissues may produce pus and any sinus tracks should be explored by probing with bacteriology swabs. Table 10.2 details some common features of ulcer types.

Investigations

Duplex ultrasonography is a cheap non-invasive method of assessing arterial and venous disease that is available in most vascular

Table 10.2 Ulcer characteristics.

Ulcer type	Location	Appearance	Associated features
Venous	Gaiter area (above malleoli)	Sloping edge Granulating base Exudate/slough	Haemosiderin skin changes Lipodermatosclerosis
Arterial	Anterior leg (shin) Over malleoli Under heel Over toe joints	Punched-out edge Grey/pale base with little granulation Typically painful	History of severe ischaemia
Neuropathic	Over malleoli Under heel Over toe joints Under metatarsal heads Medial aspect of first metatarsal head (bunion area)	Punched out Surrounding callus	Diabetes Sinus formation Underlying osteomyelitis Charcot deformity Impaired sensation

surgical clinics. It is the gold standard modality for deep and superficial venous assessment. Ultrasonographers are also able to assess arterial disease and identify flow-limiting stenoses and occlusions.

Computed tomography (CT) angiography is a widely available method of visualising peripheral arterial disease. Modern scanners are able to use low doses of contrast to image the entire vascular tree. It is limited in assessment of venous disease as it is unable to measure reflux but CT can be useful for determining causes of proximal venous obstruction (such as pelvic masses and central vein occlusion).

Magnetic resonance imaging (MRI) is an excellent method of arterial imaging and does not require the administration of contrast; however, it is of limited use in venous disease. It is more time consuming and requires greater technical expertise to produce high-quality images and is thus more expensive. MRI is especially useful to examine for evidence of osteomyelitis/deep sepsis in diabetic foot ulcer disease.

Digital subtraction angiography can be used to accurately image arterial pathology and simultaneously treat arterial stenoses and occlusions. However, it is invasive and associated with radiation exposure, risks of arterial injury/thrombosis and contrast nephropathy.

In addition to vascular investigations, haematology and standard biochemical investigations are useful as well as testing for auto-antibodies and acute and chronic markers of inflammation if an autoimmune or vasculitic aetiology is suspected.

The importance of histological examination by way of an ulcer edge biopsy cannot be ignored for 'atypical' ulcers, recalcitrant lesions and where the diagnosis remains unclear after excluding venous/arterial/diabetic aetiologies. This is a simple procedure requiring simple equipment and a local anaesthetic. Either a punch biopsy can be taken or a larger ellipse of tissue including normal skin, ulcer edge and ulcer base.

Arterial ulceration

Arterial ulcers may occur in any position on the leg (Figure 10.1). They are more common over bony prominences often related to local pressure effects. Arterial ulcers have a 'punched-out' appearance with straight sides to the ulcer edge. The base of the ulcer often appears sloughy, pale and devitalised having little or poor granulation tissue present. They often have little wound exudate and can be dry and necrotic. Infection is a common associated feature. They are often deeper than venous ulcers and involve underlying structures such as tendon or bone. The ulcer itself is usually painful. This pain is particularly noted at night or on elevation of the affected limb and is improved by placing the limb in a dependant position.

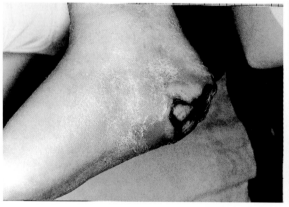

(a)

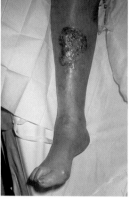

(b)

Figure 10.1 Arterial ulcers involving heel (a) and shin (b). Note associated necrosis and absence of venous skin changes.

Arterial revascularisation is the treatment for arterial ulcers. This may involve an angioplasty-based procedure. Bypass grafting in the presence of tissue loss runs a higher than average risk of serious surgical site or graft infection.

Dressings are important. Typically, these are occlusive – to allow a suitable, moist microenvironment for the growth of new tissue. They also allow the control of exudate and encourage epithelial cell migration generating an environment rich in leucocytes helping to control infection. There is also evidence that pain and pruritis are decreased by this dressing type. There is extensive current research into 'smart' active dressings that utilise nanotechonology to deliver substances such as growth factors to increase rates of healing or interact with tissue proteases to encourage epithelia activity.

Those wounds that are actively infected or carry a heavy slough load will benefit from one of the various debridement treatments available (larvae, hydrocolloid dressings, mechanical ward-based treatments or surgery). Antibacterial dressings (silver and iodine) also have a role in some instances.

Neuropathic ulceration

Neuropathy causes the loss of protective sensation and coordination of muscle groups in the foot and leg. This predisposes patients to unnoticed injuries and structural foot deformities all of which worsen repetitive stress at pressure points leading to tissue breakdown.

Diabetes is the most common cause for neuropathic ulceration, which commonly occurs on the soles of the feet particularly under the metatarsal heads (Figure 10.2). They are typically painless and are usually surrounded by callosities. The presence of sinus tracks should increase suspicion that underlying tissue and bone may be infected. Imaging with X-ray or MRI can identify underling osteomyelitis.

Often diabetic neuropathic ulcers have a degree of arterial insufficiency that also needs addressing. Only then should callus and necrotic tissue be debrided either with dressings or surgically (it is often possible to carry out extensive debridement under only

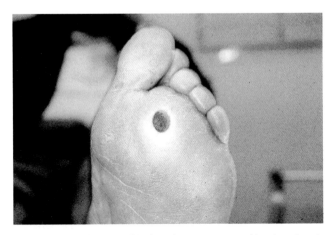

Figure 10.2 Typical neuropathic ulceration over metatarsal head on the sole of a diabetic patient's foot.

local anaesthetic because of the degree of sensory neuropathy). Any active infection should be treated to minimise the extent of possible tissue loss. The ulcerated area should then be protected with off-loading footwear or a windowed plaster cast while healing takes place.

Patients with neuropathic ulcers or feet at risk of developing diabetic ulcers should be managed along the lines of the National Service Framework for Diabetes in specialist facilities with multidisciplinary team input.

Venous ulceration

Venous hypertension is the commonest cause of leg ulceration in the Western world. This condition alone places a significant burden on NHS resources, especially considering the plethora of community-based dressings and bandages used as well as nursing time required. While community-based management based on effective compression therapy has been the traditional method of treatment, clinical trials are currently assessing the efficacy of more interventional approaches. It is important to recognise that because venous disease is so common (up to 50% of the population), it is not unusual for venous ulcers to develop in association with other contributory factors such as arterial disease and diabetes.

Venous ulcers classically develop in the medial gaiter region above the ankle usually in association with the clinical features of underlying CVI (Figure 10.3) and sometimes visible varicose veins. However, they can also be found laterally located or atypically on the foot (Figure 10.4). Patients often describe having had ulceration for protracted periods of time, sometimes decades, and a pattern of intermittent healing and recurrence is common. The clinical appearance is characterised by a superficial defect with sloping edges and florid, friable granulation tissue in the base. Venous ulcers are often associated with variable levels of slough formation and can exude large volumes of fluid. This fluid loss is often difficult to control and may cause secondary damage to surrounding skin due to the maceration that can occur. Traditionally, ulceration has been considered a consequence of previous deep vein thrombosis but assessment with duplex ultrasound scanning demonstrates that over 60% of the patients with venous ulcers have isolated superficial reflux in isolation with normal deep veins and only 1 in 10 limbs demonstrate evidence of post-thrombotic deep vein changes.

Community-based compression therapy is the cornerstone treatment modality in the United Kingdom. A systematic review and meta-analysis in 2009 demonstrated that four-layer bandaging increased the chances of ulcer healing by 30% compared with short-stretch bandaging. Previous studies have demonstrated the efficacy of superficial venous surgery in achieving ulcer healing. Prevention of recurrence of venous ulceration can be significantly enhanced by correction of superficial venous reflux in combination with compression (ESCHAR study). Currently, newer modalities of superficial venous treatment (ultrasound-guided foam sclerotherapy and thermal endovenous ablation) are being evaluated to test the efficacy of compression alone versus compression plus endovenous ablation of superficial reflux. To this end, the results of the EVRA (early venous reflux ablation) ulcer trial are awaited.

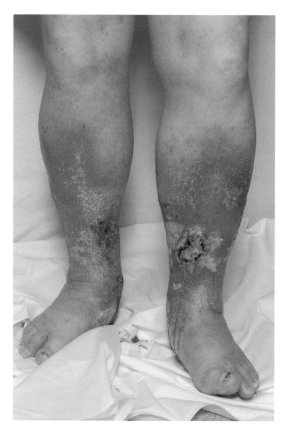

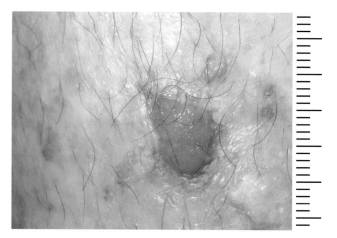

Figure 10.5 Pretibial basal cell carcinoma. Consideration of malignant lesions requires a high degree of suspicion. This lesion had shown some signs of reduction in size with community-based compression bandaging but does not demonstrate the expected features of underlying CVI.

Figure 10.3 Typical skin changes of chronic venous insufficiency demonstrating haemosiderin pigmentation, 'inverted champagne bottle legs' and bilateral ulceration over the medial gaiter region.

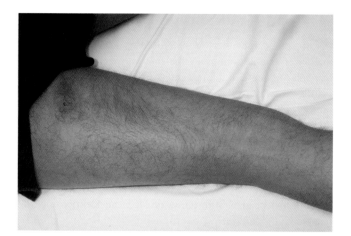

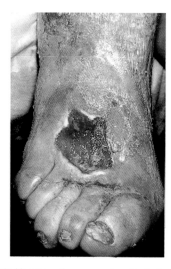

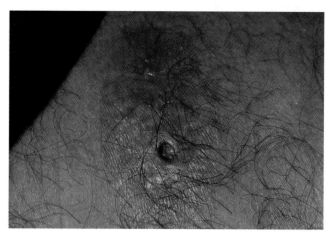

Figure 10.4 Atypical location of a venous ulcer; illustrating the requirement for full clinical assessment of lower limb ulceration to direct appropriate treatment.

Figure 10.6 Atypical tuberculous thigh ulcer.

For the majority of patients with venous ulceration, appropriate investigation and treatment can result in a healed limb; however, ulcer recurrence remains a problem and the prevention of recurrence remains an important aspect of ulcer management. Below knee class II compression hosiery (which delivers 18–24 mmHg pressure at the ankle) is effective in preventing re-ulceration in compliant patients. Many patients with venous ulcers are elderly, arthritic and find donning and doffing hosiery difficult. In these circumstances, class I (14–17 mmHg) may be a pragmatic compromise or alternative stockings with zip fasteners/wrap around designs may be more appropriate.

Timely vascular surgical referral for formal assessment of ulcers is recommended. The Venous Forum of the Royal Society of Medicine recommends that all breaks in the skin below the knee of more than 2-week duration be referred urgently to a vascular surgical department. However, despite timely and appropriate treatment, there remains a small proportion of patients (approximately 10%) with venous leg ulcers that remain unhealed after several years of treatment.

Arteriovenous ulceration

Up to 20% of leg ulcers develop as a result of combined arterial (ABPI < 0.8) and venous insufficiency (duplex evidence of venous reflux). This group of patients can be challenging as standard compression bandages are not suitable in the presence of arterial disease. Modified or reduced compression can be used with ABPI > 0.7 but in most cases correction of the arterial disease is required. This will allow the safe application of effective compression or treatment of superficial venous reflux.

Other conditions to consider

While most patients presenting with lower limb ulceration will have either venous, arterial, mixed or neuropathic ulcers occasionally, less common causes of ulceration occur (Table 10.1). These alternative diagnoses are important to make so that appropriate management can be instituted. The clinical history and examination will often alert the clinician to less typical forms of ulceration, especially if further assessment excludes arterial or venous disease. Basal cell (Figure 10.5) and squamous carcinoma are commonly confirmed on biopsy of the ulcer edge. Figure 10.6 demonstrates a thigh ulcer in an Asian patient with cutaneous TB. Patients whose ulcers develop without any obvious aetiology need careful assessment for underlying vasculitis, blood dyscrasias, rheumatoid disease, etc. before being labelled as factitious.

Clinical scenario: a patient with lower leg skin breakdown

Presentation: A 73-year-old male was referred by his GP with skin breakdown of his right lower leg. This started 5 months ago and was slowly deteriorating. The ulcer was painful and not healing with regular dressings and antibiotics for cellulitis. There was no history of trauma or previous DVT (deep venous thrombosis). He was a smoker and had borderline diabetes mellitus.

Examination findings: He had multiple areas of superficial skin breakdown in the gaiter area of right leg (with associated skin redness and haemosiderosis), as well as ulceration of a couple of toes. There were no associated varicose veins. The foot was hyperaemic looking but cold to touch and the femoral pulse was weak (and absent distal pulses).

Differential diagnosis: venous ulceration, arterial insufficiency or mixed arterial and venous disease.

Investigations: Blood tests (to exclude anaemia and significant infection), U&Es, blood sugar (HbA1c), ABPI and venous duplex scan.

Results: Blood tests were essentially normal. ABPI was reduced at 0.68 and venous duplex was normal. On the basis of the low ABPI, an arterial duplex scan was performed that revealed a tight right external iliac artery stenosis as well as stenosis in the mid thigh SFA (superficial femoral artery).

Management: He was started on aspirin and statin therapy. He underwent angioplasty of the above stenoses and the ulcers then healed over the next 3 months.

Further reading

Bailey & Love's short practice of surgery, 23rd edn. 2010.

Barwell JR, Davies CE, Deacon J *et al.* Comparison of surgery and compression with compression alone in chronic venous ulceration (ESCHAR study): randomised controlled trial. *Lancet* 2004;**363**:1854–1859.

Negus D (ed). *Leg ulcers: a practical approach to management*, 2nd edn. Butterworth Heinemann, London, 1992.

O'Mera S, Tierney J, Cullum N *et al.* Four layer bandage compared with short stretch bandage for venous leg ulcers: systematic review and meta-analysis of randomised controlled trials with data from individual patients. *BMJ* 2009;**338**:1054–1057.

Scriven JM, Hartshorne T, Bell PRF *et al.* Single-visit venous ulcer assessment clinic: the first year. *Br J Surg* 1997;**84**:334–336.

Venous Forum of the Royal Society of Medicine. Recommendations for the referral and treatment of patients with lower limb chronic venous insufficiency (including Varicose Veins). *Phlebology* 2011;**26**(3):91–93.

CHAPTER 11

Lymphoedema

Vaughan L. Keeley and Ruth A. England

Royal Derby Hospital, UK

OVERVIEW

- Lymphoedema is more common than was once thought
- Although the condition is incurable, patients can usually be helped by a combination of physical treatments
- To date, there is no effective drug treatment
- Cellulitis is an important complication that should be treated promptly with antibiotics.

Introduction

Lymphoedema is a swelling of the tissues as a result of a failure of lymphatic drainage. When it first develops, the swelling is mainly due to the accumulation of fluid, but over time fibrosis occurs and adipose tissue is deposited. In the past, lymphoedema has been considered to be uncommon and untreatable. However, current thinking is rather different, as described here.

Lymphoedema/chronic oedema

All oedema arises from an imbalance of capillary filtration and lymphatic drainage (Box 11.1). Therefore, technically, all oedema has a lymphatic component.

Box 11.1 **Factors causing lymphoedema/chronic oedema**

Factors causing an increased capillary filtration

- Increased venous pressure, e.g. in venous disease, deep vein thrombosis, heart failure, immobility
- Increased capillary pressure due to arteriolar dilation, e.g. angioedema, and drugs, e.g. nifedipine
- Reduced plasma oncotic pressure, e.g. in hypoalbuminaemia

Factors causing reduced lymphatic drainage

- Structural damage to lymphatic vessels, e.g. due to surgery and/or radiotherapy

---

- Developmental abnormality in lymphatic vessels, e.g. hypoplasia in Milroy's disease
- Reduced 'muscle pump' activity in immobility

For example, in venous disease, capillary filtration is increased as a result of increased venous pressure. This leads to an increase in lymphatic drainage to match it. When the transport capacity of the lymphatic system is exceeded, capillary filtration outstrips lymphatic drainage and oedema develops (high output failure of the lymphatics in a venous oedema). However, over time, the increased flow in the lymphatics declines, probably as a result of vessel damage, and a further failure of lymphatic drainage develops (lymphoedema).

In immobile patients, a chronic 'dependency' oedema of the lower limbs is often seen (armchair legs). This arises from a failure of the muscle pump in the legs to propel both blood and lymph in the veins and lymph vessels, respectively. Thus, venous pressure and therefore capillary filtration is increased and lymphatic flow is reduced, resulting in oedema.

In pure lymphoedema, lymphatic failure is of two types:

1 *Primary Lymphoedema*. This is due to a genetic abnormality of the lymphatic system.
2 *Secondary Lymphoedema*. This arises from an extrinsic process that damages a normal lymphatic system, e.g. surgery, trauma, radiotherapy or infection (cellulitis and filariasis).

In clinical practice, pure lymphoedema may be relatively uncommon, but many patients have chronic oedema that can have a lymphatic component. These patients suffer similar problems to those with pure lymphoedema. Thus, the umbrella term 'chronic oedema' is useful: both clinically to describe the range of conditions and in epidemiological studies looking at prevalence and aetiology.

Prevalence

The prevalence of oedema is not clear from the literature. 'Chronic oedema' has been defined as an oedema of greater than 3-month duration affecting any part of the body: limbs and mid-line structures, e.g. head and neck, trunk and genitalia. In a study carried out in Derby, UK, the prevalence was found to be 3.99 per 1000

ABC of Arterial and Venous Disease, Third Edition.
Edited by Tim England and Akhtar Nasim.
© 2015 John Wiley & Sons, Ltd. Published 2015 by John Wiley & Sons, Ltd.

CHAPTER 12

Vasculitis

Matthew D. Morgan[1], Stuart W. Smith[1], and Janson C.H. Leung[2]

[1]School of Immunity and Infection, College of Medical & Dental Sciences, University of Birmingham, UK
[2]Department of Renal Medicine, Royal Derby Hospital, UK

OVERVIEW

- The vasculitides are classified as primary or secondary, localised or systemic, and characterised by inflammation of blood vessels. The primary systemic vasculitides (PSVs) are usually grouped together as large, medium or small vessel diseases according to the smallest size of vessel involved

- The mainstay of treatment for most PSVs is still immunosuppression with corticosteroids and cytotoxic agents, but these drugs often cause significant morbidity

- Giant cell arteritis (GCA) is the most common form of PSV in the United Kingdom, whereas Takayasu's arteritis is the more common in Asia

- Polyarteritis nodosa (PAN) is rare in the United Kingdom, a disease of medium-sized arteries that leads to ischaemia or infarction within affected organs. Diagnosis is based on the demonstration of arterial aneurysms in the renal, splanchnic, hepatic or splenic vessels using angiography

- For non-hepatitis B-associated PAN, the severity of disease at presentation predicts the long-term outcome, with poorer survival seen in patients having more severe disease

- The most serious feature of Kawasaki disease (KD) is coronary artery disease; aneurysms occur in a fifth of untreated patients and may lead to myocardial infarction

- Small vessel vasculitis associated with anti-neutrophil cytoplasmic antibodies (ANCAs) may present with non-specific symptoms, e.g. fever, malaise, arthralgia, myalgia and weight loss. Once lower respiratory tract or renal disease develops, the course is usually rapidly progressive

- Granulomatosis with polyangiitis (Wegener's) (GPA), microscopic polyangiitis (MPA) and eosinophilic granulomatosis with polyangiitis (Churg–Strauss) (EGPA) have distinct features

- IgA (immunoglobulin A) vasculitis or Henoch–Schönlein purpura (HSP) is mainly a disease of children and is usually self-limiting, requiring nothing more than supportive care. The typical features comprise purpura over the buttocks and lower limbs, haematuria, abdominal pain, bloody diarrhoea and arthralgia

- C1q vasculitis or hypocomplementaemic urticarial vasculitis syndrome (HUVS) is a rare form of vasculitis characterised by generalised urticaria with persistent hypocomplementaemia

- Patients with the less common forms of systemic vasculitis or with complex or therapy-resistant disease should be managed by or in conjunction with a specialist centre with the appropriate experience.

The vasculitides are a group of diseases causing inflammation in blood vessel walls. They are usually classified as primary or secondary (to diseases such as bacterial endocarditis, systemic lupus erythematosus or drugs such as propylthiouracil) and can be localised (affecting usually only the skin or a single organ system) or systemic (affecting multiple organ systems). This chapter focuses on the primary systemic vasculitides (PSVs). The PSVs are usually grouped together as large, medium or small vessel diseases according to the smallest size of vessel involved (Figure 12.1).

The aetiopathogenesis is still not well understood for most PSVs, and so the classification of the diseases is not completely satisfactory. Most PSVs have classification criteria that were defined at the Chapel Hill Consensus Conference (CHCC). These classification criteria are based on a combination of clinical features and pathological findings. The CHCC classification criteria will be used throughout this chapter.

The clinical features seen in PSVs can be divided into those features that are common to most systemic inflammatory diseases (fever, malaise, weight loss, night sweats, arthralgia and myalgia) and those features that are specific to the organ systems involved in the disease. Evidence of an acute phase response is common to most active PSVs, with a raised serum C-reactive protein (CRP) and erythrocyte sedimentation rate (ESR) or plasma viscosity (PV).

Because the pathogenesis is still poorly understood, the mainstay of treatment for most PSVs is still immunosuppression with corticosteroids and cytotoxic agents. Many of the immunosuppressive regimes used in PSVs are associated with considerable morbidity and mortality. Many of the drug trials in recent years have been designed to investigate therapeutic regimes that reduce the immunosuppressive burden for patients while still maintaining disease control.

ABC of Arterial and Venous Disease, Third Edition.
Edited by Tim England and Akhtar Nasim.
© 2015 John Wiley & Sons, Ltd. Published 2015 by John Wiley & Sons, Ltd.

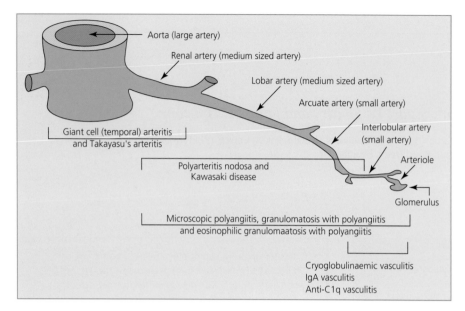

Figure 12.1 Spectrum of systemic vasculitides organised according to predominant size of vessels affected. Source: Adapted from Jennette *et al.* (2012). Reproduced with permission from John Wiley and Sons.

Large-vessel vasculitis

Giant cell arteritis (temporal arteritis)

Giant cell arteritis (GCA) is the most common form of PSV in the United Kingdom. It may affect any of the major branches of the aorta. Clinical features include unilateral throbbing headache, facial pain and claudication of the jaw when eating (Box 12.1). Visual loss is a feared complication of the disease, and it may be sudden and painless, affecting some or all of the visual field. Diplopia and other cranial nerve lesions may occur.

Box 12.1 **Definitions of large-vessel vasculitis**

GCA (temporal arteritis)

- Granulomatous arteritis of aorta and its major branches, especially extracranial branches of carotid artery
- Often affects temporal artery
- Usually occurs in patients older than 50 years
- Often associated with polymyalgia rheumatica

Takayasu's arteritis

- Granulomatous inflammation of aorta and its major branches
- Usually occurs in patients younger than 50 years

Initial treatment is with high-dose prednisolone (40–60 mg/day), which should be started as soon as the diagnosis is suspected to avoid visual loss. The diagnosis is confirmed by biopsy of the affected artery (Figure 12.2). The addition of methylprednisolone may improve remission rates and reduce corticosteroid exposure. Duplex sonography, high-resolution MRI (magnetic resonance imaging) and positron emission tomography (PET) may be useful in the initial assessment of disease extent and monitoring of vascular inflammation. The corticosteroid dose may be reduced to 10 mg/day over 6 months and then more slowly to a maintenance of 5–10 mg/day. However, a sizable number of GCA patients flare upon tapering or withdrawing corticosteroid therapy. Maintenance treatment may be required for 2 years. From the result of

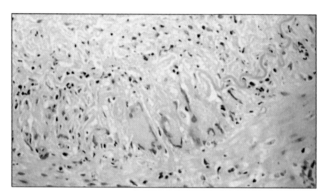

Figure 12.2 Temporal artery biopsy specimen with giant cell inflammation.

meta-analysis of three randomised control trials, the addition of methotrexate to corticosteroids may reduce risk of first relapse by 35% and the risk of second relapse by 35%, as well as corticosteroid exposure. Etanercept may also allow a reduction of corticosteroid dose for patients with side effects, but the result from one trial was not statistically significant probably due to the small sample size. The reports of use of tocilizumab, a humanised anti-interleukin 6 (IL-6) receptor antibody, are encouraging, and randomised controlled trials are needed to confirm its efficacy. Prevention of platelet aggregation with low-dose aspirin is potentially effective in preventing ischaemic complications of GCA. The disease is monitored by measuring acute phase response markers and sometimes using non-invasive imaging (Figure 12.3).

Takayasu's arteritis

Takayasu's arteritis (Box 12.1) is most common in Asia, affects more women than men and is usually diagnosed in patients <50 years of age. Inflammation and then scarring of the aorta and its major branches leads to aortic arch syndrome with claudication of the arm, loss of pulses, variation of blood pressure of >10 mmHg between the arms, arterial bruits, angina, aortic valve regurgitation, syncope, stroke and visual disturbance. Involvement of the descending aorta

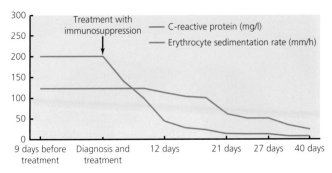

Figure 12.3 C-reactive protein concentration (>10 mg/l) and erythrocyte sedimentation rate (>18 mm/h) are raised at time of diagnosis of giant cell arteritis but fall to normal levels after starting immunosuppression therapy.

may cause bowel ischaemia, mesenteric angina, renovascular hypertension, renal impairment and lower limb claudication. Diagnosis is by angiography, MRI or PET scanning. (18)Fluorodeoxyglucose PET ((18)F-FDG_PET) is a promising new imaging technique for early diagnosis and disease monitoring. Treatment of acute disease in patients with high CRP or ESR is with corticosteroids. Cytotoxic drugs such as cyclophosphamide can be added if steroids alone do not control the disease. Encouraging preliminary results have been obtained with tocilizumab. There are case reports of successful treatments with rituximab, a monoclonal anti-CD20 antibody, and leflunomide. Surgery or angioplasty may be required for stenoses once active inflammation has been controlled.

Medium vessel vasculitis

Polyarteritis nodosa

Polyarteritis nodosa (PAN) (Box 12.2) is rare in the United Kingdom. It is associated with hepatitis B virus (HBV) infection in some patients. Disease of medium-sized arteries leads to ischaemia or infarction within affected organs. The disease can involve the gut, causing abdominal pain, bleeding or perforation; in the heart, it can cause angina or myocardial infarction; cortical infarcts and ischaemia in the kidneys can lead to renal impairment and hypertension and involvement of the peripheral nervous system can cause mononeuritis multiplex.

Diagnosis is based on the demonstration of arterial aneurysms in the renal, splanchnic, hepatic or splenic vessels using angiography (Figure 12.4). Biopsy of affected muscles or nerves may reveal histological evidence of arteritis.

> **Box 12.2 Definitions of medium-sized vessel vasculitis**
>
> Polyarteritis nodosa
> - Necrotising inflammation of medium and small arteries without glomerulonephritis, pulmonary capillaritis or disease of arterioles, capillaries or venules
>
> Kawasaki disease
> - Arteritis affecting large, medium and small arteries and associated with mucocutaneous lymph node syndrome
> - Coronary arteries are usually affected and aorta and veins maybe affected
> - Usually occurs in children

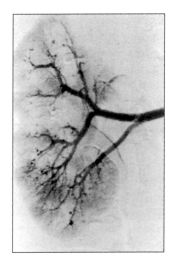

Figure 12.4 Renal angiogram showing multiple arterial aneurysms.

Treatment of PAN associated with HBV requires an antiviral drug such as interferon α or lamivudine combined with short-course, high-dose corticosteroids and plasma exchange. For non-HBV-associated PAN, the severity of disease at presentation predicts the long-term outcome, with worse survival seen in those patients having more severe disease. The addition of 12 pulses of intravenous cyclophosphamide over 10 months to corticosteroids may improve outcomes for patients with severe disease.

Kawasaki disease

Kawasaki disease (KD) (Box 12.2) was first described in Japan in 1967. It is the most common cause of acquired heart disease in children in the developed world. KD usually affects children under the age of 12. The typical clinical features are described in Box 12.3. The most serious feature of KD is coronary artery disease; aneurysms occur in one-fifth of untreated patients and may lead to myocardial infarction. They can be detected by echocardiography and, in severe circumstances, coronary reperfusion strategies are required.

> **Box 12.3 Features of mucocutaneous lymph node syndrome in Kawasaki disease**
>
> At least five features must be present
> - Fever for >5 days
> - Conjunctival congestion
> - Changes to lips and oral cavity: dry, red, fissured lips; strawberry tongue; reddening of oral and pharyngeal mucosa
> - Changes of peripheral extremities: red palms and soles; indurative oedema; desquamation of finger tips during convalescence
> - Macular polymorphous rash on trunk
> - Swollen cervical lymph nodes

The aetiology of KD remains unknown, with clinical and epidemiologic data suggesting an unknown infective cause. Recently, an antigen-driven IgA response directed at cytoplasmic inclusion bodies in KD-affected tissues was identified. Light and microscopic studies showed that the inclusion bodies are consistent with aggregates of viral protein and RNA and were probably formed by the unknown KD infectious aetiologic agent.

Treatments include high-dose intravenous immunoglobulins (IVIgs) that reduce the prevalence of coronary artery aneurysms, provided that treatment is started within 10 days of onset of the disease. Low-dose aspirin is recommended for thrombocythaemia. A recent study in a Japanese population of KD patients at high risk of IVIg resistance found that the addition of corticosteroids to aspirin and IVIG may reduce the incidence of coronary artery aneurysms. Anti-TNFα therapy, infliximab, has been investigated in small open label studies and may be useful in children with refractory or resistant disease. Children with persistent or remodelled coronary aneurysms after KD have a high rate of complications including thrombosis or stenosis leading to myocardial infarction. It is not clear whether patients with KD are at risk of accelerated atherosclerosis.

Small vessel vasculitis associated with anti-neutrophil cytoplasmic antibodies

The early symptoms of these disorders are non-specific, with fever, malaise, arthralgia, myalgia and weight loss, and patients in whom such symptoms are persistent should be screened for anti-neutrophil cytoplasmic antibodies (ANCAs), have their ESR and CRP concentration measured and have their urine tested for blood with a dipstick. Early diagnosis is essential to prevent potentially life-threatening renal and pulmonary injury. Delays in diagnosis are unfortunately common, and this often leads to serious morbidity. Once respiratory or renal disease develops, the course is usually rapidly progressive.

Granulomatosis with polyangiitis (Wegener's granulomatosis)

Upper respiratory tract disease occurs in >90% of cases of granulomatosis with polyangiitis (GPA, previously known as Wegener's granulomatosis). Lung disease is common, with cough, haemoptysis and dyspnoea, and may progress to life-threatening pulmonary haemorrhage.

The kidneys are affected in up to 80% of cases; blood, protein and casts are present in the urine and should be examined by dipstick testing and microscopy. If untreated, there is loss of renal function, often within days. Other features include purpuric rashes, nail fold infarcts and ocular manifestations including conjunctival haemorrhages, scleritis, uveitis, keratitis, proptosis or ocular muscle paralysis due to retro-orbital inflammation. The disease can affect the gut, causing haemorrhage, the heart, causing coronary artery ischaemia, and the neurological system, causing sensory neuropathy or mononeuritis multiplex. The two pathological hallmarks of GPA are chronic granulomatous inflammation and vasculitis. Granulomas in the lung may coalesce into large masses that cavitate, mimicking tumours (Figure 12.5).

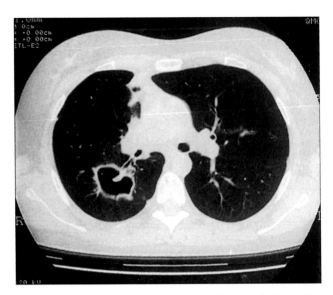

Figure 12.5 Cavitating granulomatous lesion in right lung of patient with granulomatosis with polyangiitis.

Microscopic polyangiitis (microscopic polyarteritis)

Microscopic polyangiitis (MPA) has many similarities to GPA, but disease of the upper respiratory tract is uncommon in MPA, although pulmonary haemorrhage may occur. Patients with MPA usually have glomerulonephritis, and, rarely, disease may be limited to the kidney. No granuloma formation is seen.

Diagnosis

Diagnosis is based on typical clinical features, tissue biopsy and the presence of ANCAs (Box 12.4). Sometimes, ANCA tests are negative, particularly if disease is limited to the upper respiratory tract (Table 12.1). Antibody titres usually fall and may disappear completely when the disease is in remission.

Box 12.4 **Definitions for classification of vasculitides often associated with anti-neutrophil cytoplasmic antibodies**

Granulomatosis with polyangiitis

- Granulomatous inflammation of the respiratory tract
- Necrotising vasculitis affecting small to medium-sized vessels (capillaries, venules, arterioles and arteries)
- Necrotising glomerulonephritis is common

Microscopic polyangiitis

- Necrotising vasculitis with few or no immune deposits affecting small vessels (capillaries, venules, arterioles and arteries)
- Necrotising arteritis of small and medium-sized arteries may be present
- Necrotising glomerulonephritis is very common
- Pulmonary capillaritis often occurs

Eosinophilic granulomatosis with polyangiitis

- Eosinophil-rich and granulomatous inflammation of respiratory tract
- Necrotising vasculitis affecting small to medium-sized vessels
- Blood eosinophilia ($>1.5 \times 10^9$/l)
- Usually associated with asthma

Table 12.1 Specificity and sensitivity of ANCA serology testing for granulomatosis with polyangiitis (Wegener's granulomatosis) and microscopic polyangiitis.

	Specificity/sensitivity (%)
Specificity of assays (related to disease controls)	
Indirect immunofluorescence	
cANCA	95
pANCA	81
ELISAs	
PR3-ANCA	87
MPO-ANCA	91
Combined indirect immunofluorescence and ELISA	
cANCA/PR3-ANCA positive	99
pANCA/MPO-ANCA positive	99
Sensitivity of combined testing	
Wegener's granulomatosis	73
Microscopic polyangiitis	67

Source: Hagen *et al.* (1998). Reproduced by permission of Nature Publishing Group.

Treatment

Treatment of GPA and MPA comprises induction of remission and then maintenance of remission. The intensity of immunosuppression should be determined by the severity of the disease (Box 12.5). For moderate and severe disease, induction treatment should comprise cyclophosphamide and prednisolone, with the addition of methylprednisolone and/or plasma exchange for patients with severe disease. Rituximab has emerged as an alternative induction therapy to cyclophosphamide for patients with GPA and MPA, particularly for patients in whom the side effects of cyclophosphamide are unacceptable (e.g. premature menopause in women and male infertility). Patients with mild and limited disease may respond to methotrexate with prednisolone, although response rates are less good. Once induction therapy is finished, patients typically go on to maintenance therapy of variable doses of azathioprine and prednisolone. Relapses occur in 40–50% of patients during the first 5 years, so lifelong monitoring for recurring disease activity is essential.

Box 12.5 **Treatment of ANCA-associated small vessel vasculitis**

Induction therapy (minimum 3 months from diagnosis)

- Oral cyclophosphamide (2 mg/kg with dose reduction for age and renal impairment)
- Or Intravenous cyclophosphamide at weeks 0, 2 and 4 and every 3 weeks thereafter (maximum 10 pulses)
- Or Rituximab 375 mg/m^2 weekly × 4 doses or 1 g fortnightly for 2 doses

---

Pulsed i.v. cyclophosphamide dose reduction for renal function and age

Age (years)	Creatinine (µmol/l)	
	<300	**>300**
<60	15 mg/kg/pulse	12.5 mg/kg/pulse
>60 and <70	12.5 mg/kg/pulse	10 mg/kg/pulse
>70	10 mg/kg/pulse	7.5 mg/kg/pulse

CYCLOPS regimen, adapted from Harper *et al.* (2012).

- Prednisolone 1 mg/kg/day (maximum 80 mg) reducing to 12.5 mg/day at 4 months
- For patients with severe disease or life-threatening disease (severe crescentic glomerulonephritis with creatinine >500 µmol/l or pulmonary haemorrhage), consider the addition of three pulses of methylprednisolone 15 mg/kg/day for 3 days and/or plasma exchange, 7–10 treatments over 14 days
- For patients with persistent disease despite cyclophosphamide therapy, consider switching to rituximab

Maintenance therapy (minimum of 18 months, longer if clinically indicated)

- Azathioprine 2 mg/kg/day (maximum 200 mg/day); reduce dose by 25 mg/day if age >60 years
- Prednisolone 5 mg/day

Relapse therapy

- Major relapse: return to induction therapy and consider rituximab to limit cyclophosphamide exposure
- Minor relapse: temporarily increase dose of corticosteroids

Cautions

- Stop cyclophosphamide or azathioprine if white blood count $<4 \times 10^9$/l; restart with a dose reduction of 25% once white blood count $>4 \times 10^9$/l
- Consider gastric and bone protection; consider fungal and *Pneumocystis jirovecii* prophylaxis (for both cyclophosphamide and rituximab induction therapies)
- Consider bladder protection when using intravenous cyclophosphamide (mesna)

Eosinophilic granulomatosis with polyangiitis (Churg–Strauss syndrome)

Eosinophilic granulomatosis with polyangiitis (EGPA, previously known as Churg–Strauss syndrome) is associated with an atopic tendency, usually asthma. Patients not infrequently present with peripheral neuropathy or mononeuritis multiplex. It may also affect coronary, pulmonary, cerebral and splanchnic circulations. Rashes with purpura, urticaria and subcutaneous nodules are common. Glomerulonephritis may develop, but renal failure is uncommon. Diagnosis depends on the presence of typical clinical features, biopsy of skin, lung and kidney and blood eosinophilia. ANCA was only detected in 30–40% of patients. Patients without poor prognostic features may respond adequately to corticosteroids alone;

those patients with poor prognostic features require additional immunosuppression usually with cyclophosphamide. The optimal length of immunosuppression for EGPA has not been established, and relapse rates remain high. Asthma requires conventional treatment, but leucotriene receptor antagonist drugs have been causally linked with EGPA and should be avoided in these patients.

Small vessel vasculitis without anti-neutrophil cytoplasmic antibodies

Immunoglobulin a vasculitis (Henoch–Schönlein purpura)

Immunoglobulin A vasculitis [IgA vasculitis, also known as Henoch–Schönlein purpura (HSP)] (Box 12.6) is mainly a disease of children (2–33 times more common in children) and is usually self-limiting, requiring nothing more than supportive care. In children, it is more common in autumn and winter and frequently occurs after an upper respiratory tract infection. In adults, there is an association of IgA vasculitis with malignancies. The typical features comprise purpura over the buttocks and lower limbs (Figure 12.6), haematuria, abdominal pain, bloody diarrhoea and arthralgia. The pathological hallmarks are deposition of IgA at the dermo-epidermal junction and within the glomerular mesangium, with a mesangial hypercellular glomerulonephritis. Some patients develop a glomerular lesion resembling that seen in ANCA associated vasculitis. The renal disease may occur in isolation without any other typical manifestations. Bowel involvement can cause severe bleeding and intussusception, and renal involvement with the development of nephritis can result in renal failure. Prednisolone early in the course of the disease may reduce the abdominal pain and time to resolution of symptoms. However, there is no evidence that early corticosteroid use will prevent renal disease in patients with IgA vasculitis. Children with IgA vasculitis nephritis and persistent proteinuria $>0.5\,g/day$ per $1.73\,m^2$ should be treated with ACE (angiotensin-converting-enzyme) inhibition first. If proteinuria persists despite ACE inhibition with proteinuria $>1\,g/day$ per $1.73\,m^2$ and $GFR > 50\,ml/min$ per $1.73\,m^2$, a 6-month course of corticosteroid should be considered. IgA vasculitis nephritis in adults should be treated as in children. If crescents

are present in more than 50% of glomeruli on renal biopsy with either nephrotic syndrome or rapidly deteriorating renal function clinically, treatment with cyclophosphamide and steroid should be considered.

Box 12.6 Definitions of non-ANCA-associated small vessel vasculitis

IgA vasculitis (HSP)

- Vasculitis with IgA-dominant immune deposits affecting small vessels (capillaries, venules or arterioles)
- Affects skin, gut and glomeruli
- Associated with arthralgia or arthritis

Cryoglobulinaemic vasculitis (mixed essential cryoglobulinaemia)

- Vasculitis with cryoglobulin immune deposits affecting small vessels
- Associated with cryoglobulins in serum
- Skin and glomeruli often affected

Anti-C1q vasculitis (hypocomplementaemic urticarial vasculitis syndrome, HUVS)

- Diffuse urticarial exanthema
- Low serum complements and presence of anti-C1q antibodies
- Affects skin, joints, eyes, lung, larynx and glomeruli

Isolated cutaneous leucocytoclastic vasculitis

- Isolated cutaneous leucocytoclastic angiitis without systemic vasculitis or glomerulonephritis
- May evolve into systemic vasculitis

Cryoglobulinaemic vasculitis (mixed, essential)

Cryoglobulins are immunoglobulins that precipitate in the cold. The mixed cryoglobulin consists of a monoclonal IgM rheumatoid factor complexed to polyclonal IgG. Vasculitis (Box 12.6) develops when cryoglobulins deposit in blood vessels. Mixed essential cryoglobulinaemia is due to hepatitis C virus (HCV) infection in >80% of cases. Other causes of cryoglobulinaemia include dysproteinaemias, autoimmune diseases and chronic infections. The concentrations of serum complements C4 and C3 are reduced. Clinical features include palpable purpura, arthralgia, distal necroses, peripheral neuropathy, abdominal pain and glomerulonephritis (Figure 12.7).

The evidence base for treatment of cryoglobulinaemia with or without HCV is still limited. The majority of case series in the literature support the use of a combination of interferons with or without ribavarin, and more recently anti-virals such as protease inhibitors boceprevir and telaprevir, to suppress HCV replication, and some form of immunosuppression. Steroids and cyclophosphamide have been widely used to suppress antibody formation and inflammation in acute disease, although this may be poorly tolerated and lead to increased viral load. Plasma exchange is widely used to remove circulating autoantibodies. Several studies have demonstrated that rituximab may be effective when cryoglobulinaemic vasculitis is refractory to antiviral regimen, and the use of rituximab together with antiviral treatment may induce a better and faster clinical remission.

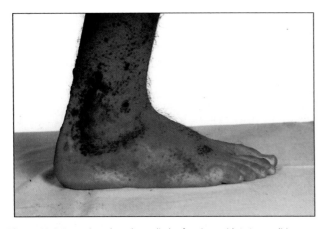

Figure 12.6 Purpuric rash on lower limb of patient with IgA vasculitis (Henoch–Schönlein purpura).

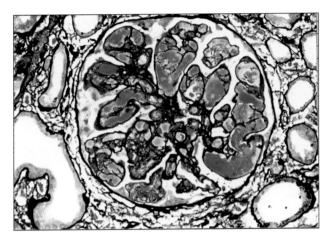

Figure 12.7 Renal biopsy specimen showing intraglomerular deposit of cryoglobulins.

Anti-C1q vasculitis (hypocomplementaemic urticarial vasculitis syndrome)

Anti-C1q vasculitis or HUVS is characterised by generalised urticaria with persistent hypocomplementaemia. It is very rare, and with the peak incidence in the fifth decade of life. Major diagnostic criteria of anti-C1q vasculitis include chronic urticarial exanthema and hypocomplementaemia; minor criteria include leucocytoclastic vasculitis, arthritis and arthralgia, glomerulonephritis, uveitis or episcleritis, abdominal pain and positive anti-C1q antibody. Angioedema, laryngeal oedema and chronic obstructive lung disease may also be present. Typical laboratory findings include low complement levels of classical pathway, namely, C1q, C3 and C4, raised ESR, anti-C1q antibodies and positive antinuclear antibodies (ANA) without anti-double-stranded DNA. The main differential diagnoses are systemic lupus erythromatosis (SLE) and cryoglobulinaemic vasculitis. Treatment is determined by severity of disease. It typically involves corticosteroids. Other immunosuppressive agents have also demonstrated some success in single cases or small case series but the rarity of disease means that there is very little evidence to support use of any single agent.

Isolated cutaneous leucocytoclastic vasculitis

This condition (Box 12.6) is often associated with a drug hypersensitivity response and improves when the drug is stopped. Occasional patients may require corticosteroids for severe disease.

Anti-glomerular basement membrane antibody-mediated disease (Goodpasture's disease)

No CHCC definition exists for this rare disease. The hallmarks are a rapidly progressive global and diffuse glomerulonephritis, as seen in small vessel vasculitides, or the presence of pulmonary haemorrhage or both. Diagnosis depends on finding antibodies to glomerular basement membrane in the serum and linear staining for IgG along the glomerular basement membrane. The antibodies, which are directed against the $\alpha3$-chain of type IV collagen, have been implicated in disease pathogenesis. About 15–30% of patients

have detectable ANCAs. Treatment is with cyclophosphamide and steroids with the addition of plasma exchange to remove circulating antibodies. There is a low probability of recovery of renal function once patients are dialysis dependent, and treatment may be less intensive for this group of patients if there is no evidence of lung involvement.

Clinical scenario: a case of pulmonary-renal syndrome

Presentation: A 29-year-old man presented to the MAU with sudden onset of haemoptysis. Preceding this he has a 4-week history of increasing tiredness, joint pain and shortness of breath. He has no significant past medical history or any relevant family history. He is a lifelong non-smoker.

Examination: In respiratory distress, pulse rate was 120/min (regular), BP was 160/90, respiratory rate was 40/min and oxygen saturation was 88% (on air). Small nail fold infarcts were noticed on his fingers. Respiratory examination revealed crepitations bilaterally. Dipstick urine revealed 4+ blood and 3+ protein. Microscopy of urine revealed presence of red cell casts. Rest of the examination was unremarkable.

Differential diagnosis: The patient has pulmonary-renal syndrome possibly due to (i) small vessel vasculitis (GPA or MPA), (ii) anti-GBM (Goodpasture's) disease and (iii) systemic lupus erythematosus.

Investigations: (i) Blood tests (FBC, U&Es, LFTs, glucose, ANCA, anti-GBM, ANA, C3 and C4, CRP) and (ii) urgent chest X-ray and ultrasound of renal tract.

Results: Creatinine 530 µmol/L, CRP 152 mg/L, Hb 80 g/L, cANCA positive with anti-PR3 level of >100 U/ml, CXR shows bilateral alveolar shadowing compatible with pulmonary haemorrhage.

Management: Patient was admitted to renal HDU. Methylprednisolone and plasma exchange were started immediately. He underwent a kidney biopsy that showed diffuse crescentic glomerulonephritis. Intravenous cyclophosphamide was started following kidney biopsy result.

Outcome: He went home after a 14-day stay in hospital with creatinine of 150 µmol/L to return at a later date for further doses of intravenous cyclophosphamide. He is on a tapering dose of oral prednisolone.

Further reading

Chapter 11: Henoch–Schonlein purpura nephritis. *Kidney Int Suppl* 2012;**2**:218–220.

Chiche L, Bataille S, Kaplanski G *et al*. The place of immunotherapy in the management of HCV-induced vasculitis: an update. *Clin Dev Immunol* 2012;**2012**:315167.

deMenthon M and Mahr A. Treating polyarteritisnodosa: current state of the art. *Clin Exp Rheumatol* 2011;**1**(Suppl 64):S110–S116.

Dominguez SR and Anderson MS. Advances in the treatment of Kawasaki disease. *Curr Opin Pediatr* 2013;**1**:103–109.

Grotz W, Baba HA, Becker JU *et al*. Hypocomplementemic urticarial vasculitis syndrome: an interdisciplinary challenge. *Dtsch Arztebl Int* 2009;**106**:756–763.

Hagen EC, Daha MR, Hermans J *et al*. Diagnostic value of standardized assays for anti-neutrophil cytoplasmic antibodies in idiopathic systemic vasculitis. EC/BCR Project for ANCA Assay Standardization. *Kidney Int* 1998;**53**:743–753.

Harper L, Morgan MD, Walsh M *et al*. Pulse versus daily oral cyclophosphamide for induction of remission in ANCA-associated vasculitis: long-term follow-up. *Ann Rheum Dis* 2012;**71**:955–960.

Jennette JC, Falk RJ, Bacon PA *et al*. 2012 revised international Chapel Hill consensus conference nomenclature of vasculitides. *Arthritis Rheum* 2013;**65**:1–11.

Miloslavsky EM, Specks U, Merkel PA *et al*. Clinical outcomes of remission induction therapy for severe antineutrophil cytoplasmic antibody-associated vasculitis. *Arthritis Rheum* 2013;**65**:2441–2449.

Ness T, Bley TA, Schmidt WA *et al*. The diagnosis and treatment of giant cell arteritis. *Dtsch Arztebl Int* 2013;**110**:376–385.

Unizony S, Stone JH and Stone JR. New treatment strategies in large-vessel vasculitis. *Curr Opin Rheumatol* 2013;**1**:3–9.

Wen D, Du X and Ma CS. Takayasu arteritis: diagnosis, treatment and prognosis. *Int Rev Immunol* 2012;**6**:462–473.

CHAPTER 13

Vascular Anomalies

E. Kate Waters and William D. Adair

Leicester Royal Infirmary, UK

OVERVIEW

- Vascular anomalies are rare, occurring in approximately 1.5% of the population. Historically, there has been confusion over the nomenclature and classification of this diverse group of lesions
- The International Society for the Study of Vascular Anomalies (ISSVA) classification brings some clarity, separating these lesions into vascular tumours and vascular malformations (Table 13.1)
- For a quick 'rule of thumb' for determining clinical management, vascular malformations can be usefully divided into high- and low-flow lesions, dependent on their blood flow characteristics
- Vascular anomalies have clinical and imaging features that overlap with other benign and aggressive pathologies, including soft tissue sarcomas
- Treatment may involve many clinical specialties including interventional radiology, vascular or reconstructive surgery and dermatology, and patients are best managed by a multidisciplinary team.

Vascular tumours

Infantile haemangiomas (strawberry naevi) are the most common childhood vascular tumour, occurring in 12% of infants. Typically, these lesions are not visible at birth but rapidly enlarge during a proliferative phase up to the age of 6 months. Growth characteristically slows down till the age of 1 year and there is subsequent gradual involution of the lesion with complete involution in 50% of individuals at 5 years of age and in 90% of individuals at 9 years. The majority of cases will have subtle residual skin changes.

Diagnosis is usually made on clinical history and examination findings alone without the need for imaging. Infantile haemangiomas with superficial dermal components have a classic strawberry appearance (Figure 13.1), while deeper lesions not involving subcutaneous tissue can have a blue appearance.

Management of haemangioma is conservative in the majority of cases with even larger lesions naturally involuting over time. Recently, treatment with topical beta-blocker has been found to be effective for superficial lesions. Intervention is indicated if

Table 13.1 The International Society for the Study of Vascular Anomalies (ISSVA) classification of vascular anomalies.

Vascular tumours	Vascular malformations
Haemangioma	Capillary
• Infantile haemangioma	• Capillary malformation (CM)
• Congenital haemangioma	• Port wine stain
• Non-involutional congenital haemangioma (NICH)	
	Venous
	• Blue rubber bleb naevus
Tumours	• Cerebral cavernous malformation (CCM)
• Kaposiform haemangioendothelioma	• Venous malformation (VM)
• Tufted angioma	
• Pyogenic granuloma	Lymphatic
	• Lymphatic malformation (micro-/macro-cystic)
Malignant tumours	
• Angiosarcoma	Arterial
	• Arteriovenous malformation (AVM)
	• Capillary malformation-AVM
	• Hereditary haemorrhagic telangiectasia (HHT)
	Combined
	• Capillaro-venous malformation (CVM)
	• Capillaro-lymphaticovenous malformation (CLVM)
	Syndrome associated
	• Klippel–Trenaunay: port wine stain, CLVM and limb hypertrophy
	• Parkes–Weber: CLVM with AVM
	• Sturge–Weber: port wine stain and leptomeningeal angiomas

Source: Dompartin *et al.* (2010). Reproduced by permission of SAGE Publications.

complications occur such as mass effect on adjacent structures, in particular, the airway or orbits, consumptive coagulopathy (Kasabach–Merritt syndrome), ulceration and bleeding.

High output cardiac failure is a rarely occurring complication of infantile haemangioma requiring medical treatment and embolisation of the capillary bed. Other vascular tumours include congenital haemangioma, present and fully formed at birth, pyogenic granuloma and tufted angioma.

ABC of Arterial and Venous Disease, Third Edition.
Edited by Tim England and Akhtar Nasim.
© 2015 John Wiley & Sons, Ltd. Published 2015 by John Wiley & Sons, Ltd.

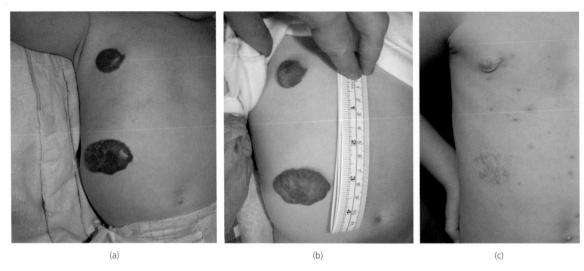

(a)   (b)   (c)

Figure 13.1 Infantile haemangioma (strawberry naevus): (a) at 5 months, (b) at 9 months and (c) at 5 years (with additional varicella).

Vascular malformations

Vascular malformations develop as a result of abnormal vessel angiogenesis. Therefore, unlike vascular tumours, they are dysplastic rather than proliferative. They are always present at birth, although they may not be clinically evident for months or years. These lesions can undergo periods of enlargement particularly during puberty, pregnancy or following trauma and do not spontaneously regress. It is usually possible to differentiate between low- and high-flow malformations on clinical history and examination. Imaging being used to confirm diagnoses and to plan any subsequent treatment (Table 13.2).

Low-flow vascular malformations
Capillary malformation

Salmon patch (erythema nuchae) and port wine stains (naevus flamus) are examples of capillary malformations (CMs). Salmon patches are very common, occurring in approximately 40% of newborns. They are red macular lesions commonly involving the nape of the neck, the upper eyelids or on the forehead between the eyebrows. They become more prominent when the infant cries or has a fever, and usually disappear by 2 years of age. Port wine stains (Figure 13.2a) occur in 0.3% of newborns and are well-demarcated purple or dark red patches most commonly affecting the face. They are usually dermatomal in distribution and unilateral, growing proportionately over time with the child. They do not regress

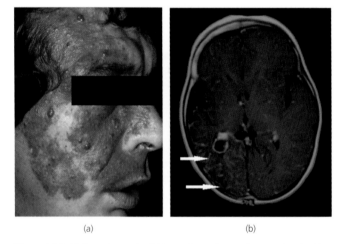

(a)   (b)

Figure 13.2 (a) Port wine stain. (b) Port wine stains can be associated with leptomeningeal vascular malformations in Sturge–Weber syndrome. Contrast-enhanced T1-weighted axial MRI demonstrates right-sided prominent leptomeningeal enhancement (arrows) of leptomeningeal haemangioma, with associated cerebral hemiatrophy.

spontaneously and can evolve from being flat to become nodular and thickened. Associated bone and soft tissue hypertrophy can occur. Port wine stains are usually an isolated abnormality, but can occur as part of the Sturge–Weber syndrome. This is the association of a capillary vascular malformation affecting one branch of the trigeminal nerve of the face, with a leptomeningeal vascular malformation and vascular malformation of the eye (Figure 13.2b).

Venous malformations

Venous malformations (VMs) consist of abnormal venous channels of varying size within a connective tissue and fatty stroma, which connect with adjacent veins. Local intravascular coagulopathy is a feature, which combined with slow venous flow makes them prone to thrombosis. Pain and swelling secondary to thrombosis are common presenting symptoms of VMs in late childhood or

Table 13.2 Classification of vascular malformations according to their flow dynamics.

High-flow vascular malformations	Low-flow vascular malformations
Arteriovenous malformations (AVMs)	Venous malformations (VMs)
	Lymphatic malformations (LMs)
	Combined malformations (CVM, CLVM)

Source: McCafferty and Jones (2011). Reproduced by permission of Elsevier.

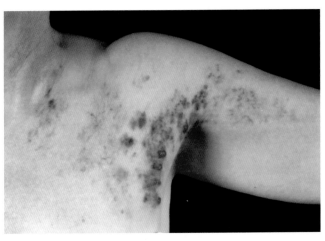

Figure 13.3 Superficial venous malformation. The blue papular parts of the lesion can be emptied with compression and spontaneously refill.

early adulthood. Symptoms may also relate to the size and site of VM. For example, those located within muscles can be painful on movement. The lesions are non-pulsatile, often with associated swelling and blue discolouration of the skin, and can be tender (Figure 13.3). They classically distend when dependent and empty on elevation of the lesion, depending on the number and integrity of the venous channels. Firm small calcified phleboliths may be palpable secondary to thrombosis. Rarely, VMs are multiple, located in the skin and visceral organs, as part of the blue rubber bleb naevus syndrome.

Lymphatic malformations

Lymphatic malformations are the second most common vascular malformation. Arising from lymphatic vessels, the majority are present at birth with 90% seen at 2 years of age. Lymphatic malformations are most commonly located in the neck, where they are often known as cystic hygromas (Figure 13.4).

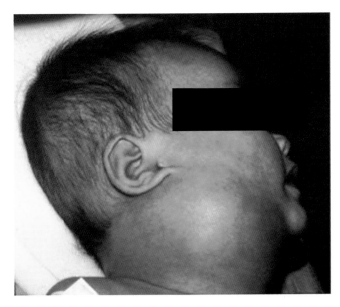

Figure 13.4 Lymphangioma (cystic hygroma).

Mixed malformations

There is considerable overlap between venous and lymphatic malformations with many lesions having various different tissue morphologies within different areas of the same malformation.

High-flow vascular malformations

An arteriovenous malformation (AVM) consists of direct connections between the arterial and venous system, bypassing the normal capillary bed of organs and tissues, and any malformation with such an arterial component is considered high flow.

AVMs are present at birth but may not become apparent until puberty or adulthood. Puberty, pregnancy and trauma can induce rapid enlargement of these lesions. The Schobinger classification of AVMs grades lesions according to symptomatology (Table 13.3). Pain, bleeding and ulceration are common presenting symptoms: high output cardiac failure is rare. Clinical examination usually reveals a warm, pulsatile mass with skin discolouration. Limb overgrowth may be noted due to hypertrophy or venous hypertension (Figure 13.5).

Imaging vascular malformations

The diagnosis of vascular anomalies is mostly through clinical assessment, but a handheld Doppler ultrasound is a useful adjunct to gauge the presence of arterial flow.

Duplex ultrasound is an accessible, non-invasive first-line investigation that can give more specific information regarding exact location, presence of vascular spaces and flow characteristics.

Magnetic Resonance Imaging (MRI) gives detailed analysis of lesions without ionising radiation and can more fully assess the extent of infiltrative and deeper lesions. MRI is also useful in evaluation of those vascular anomalies that are clinically indeterminate and can aid in their differentiation from more sinister lesions. Detailed information regarding the anatomical extent, and vascular supply, can be obtained as a prelude to treatment (Figure 13.6a and b).

Computed Tomography (CT) is not routinely used in the assessment of vascular anomalies. The radiation dose of a diagnostic CT is justified only in rare circumstances.

Catheter venography/angiography is essential for treatment planning of both low- and high-flow malformations, providing detailed

Table 13.3 Schobinger classification of arteriovenous malformation by symptoms.

Schobinger stage	Symptoms/clinical findings
I Quiescent	Stable lesion, pink/bluish stain, warmth. AV shunting seen on Doppler US
II Expanding	Type I plus enlargement, pulsations, thrill, bruit, tortuous tense veins
III Symptomatic	Type II plus pain, bleeding, ulceration, tissue necrosis, functional problems
IV Decompensating	Type III plus high output cardiac failure

Source: McCafferty and Jones (2011). Reproduced by permission of Elsevier.

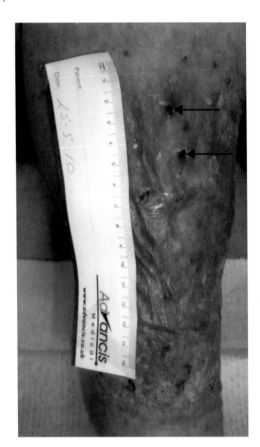

Figure 13.5 AVM within the anterior compartment of the leg. Note the skin changes secondary to venous hypertension as well as small ulcers (arrows) that presented periodically with life-threatening haemorrhage.

information about flow characteristics and feeding and draining vessels. It is usually performed during the same session as the treatment (Figure 13.7b and c).

Management of vascular malformations

Low-flow vascular malformations

There are various treatment options for low-flow vascular malformations, but the majority of patients with these lesions can be managed conservatively. The use of cosmetics and camouflage creams, analgesia for episodes of pain, venous compression stockings and antibiotics for infections associated with lymphatic malformations has a role. Avoidance of the combined oral contraceptive to reduce thrombotic risk may be appropriate. Counselling and screening for associated genetic syndromes might be required.

Venous malformations

Percutaneous sclerotherapy is the primary treatment if conservative measures have failed to manage symptoms, in particular pain. Sclerotherapy aims to obliterate the venous lumen and shrink the lesion. Following direct puncture of the venous channels using ultrasound and fluoroscopic guidance, agents such as ethanol, bleomycin or sodium tetradecyl sulphate are injected (Figure 13.6c).

Swelling and pain in the region of the malformation generally increases in the first 2 weeks post procedure, and patients must

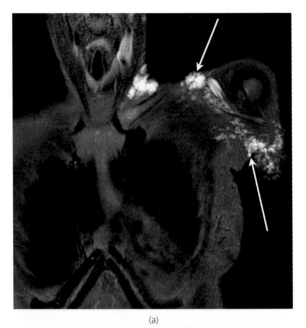

(a)

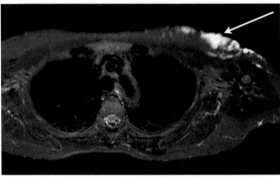

(b)

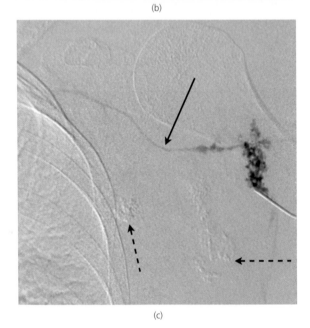

(c)

Figure 13.6 Fat saturated coronal (a) and axial (b) T2-weighted MRI sequences through the chest. The venous malformation shown in Figure 13.3 is clearly visible (arrows). (c) Venogram of venous malformation. Note draining vein (solid arrow). Two areas have been sclerosed at the same session (dotted arrows).

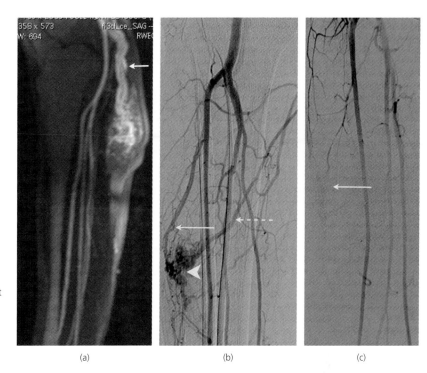

Figure 13.7 (a) MR angiogram of leg AVM (same patient as Figure 13.5). (b) Catheter angiogram: note nidus (arrowhead), major feeding artery (arrow) and draining vein (dotted arrow). (c) Catheter angiogram post embolisation with Onyx™ – note obliteration of the nidus (arrow).

(a) (b) (c)

be warned of the expected time course of symptom improvement, which can take several months. Extensive VMs may require multiple treatment sessions. Approximately 20% of the patients can expect to have complete relief of symptoms after one course of treatment, 60% should have a decrease in symptoms, while 20% receive no therapeutic benefit. Complications occur in up to 15% of the cases. These include skin necrosis and nerve damage (which can be transient). PE (pulmonary embolism), DVT (deep vein thrombosis), DIC (disseminated intravascular coagulation) and death are very rare post sclerotherapy.

Lymphatic malformations

Percutaneous sclerotherapy using a variety of sclerosants (notably bleomycin or doxycycline) can achieve satisfactory long-term outcomes, particularly in lesions with a macro-cystic component. There are difficult-to-treat subsets of lymphatic malformations that may also require surgical debulking.

High-flow vascular malformations

High-flow vascular malformations are the most difficult to treat, with high rates of recurrence and frequently occurring complications. As a result, treatment should be reserved for symptomatic lesions, i.e. Stage III and IV Schobinger classification lesions (Table 13.3). Surgical excision or debulking has limited value in the management of most AVMs, and should surgery become necessary, results are often disappointing.

Radiological embolisation is the first-line treatment choice. Peri-procedure pain from preferred agents and long procedure times necessitate general anaesthesia. Embolisation aims to obliterate the arteriovenous shunts. Various liquid embolics can be used including ethanol, sodium tetradecyl sulphate or Onyx™ (a liquid

ethylene vinyl alcohol copolymer that forms a cast on contact with blood; it has the unusual side effect of giving the patient a garlic-like odour for 24–48 h after treatment). These agents can be delivered to the AVM by transarterial or transvenous access or by direct injection into the lesion (Figure 13.7a–c).

Particulate or large embolic devices such as embolisation coils and Amplatzer plugs are rarely used, although the latter are most useful in the treatment of pulmonary AVMs, most commonly associated with hereditary haemorrhagic telangiectasia (HHT).

The majority of lesions will require more than one embolisation treatment and the patient must be consented for this. Complications are the same as for low-flow sclerotherapy but are likely to occur with increased incidence in high-flow lesions. High-flow vascular malformations have the highest rate of recurrence, particularly with insufficient or incorrect treatment of the original lesion. Each patient should be followed up for at least 2 years to detect any sign of AVM recurrence and to monitor for complications.

Conclusions

- Vascular anomalies are divided into vascular tumours and vascular malformations.
- Vascular malformations are a challenging group of conditions, best managed by a multidisciplinary team with expertise primarily from interventional radiologists and vascular surgeons as well as dermatologists and plastic surgeons.
- The diagnosis and management of these lesions is made mainly on clinical assessment, correlated with flow dynamics on Doppler ultrasound confirming the low- or high-flow nature of the lesions.
- MRI can be useful to confirm the diagnosis, exclude other pathologies, and plan treatment where necessary.

- The majority of vascular malformations can be managed conservatively. Treatment is reserved for those with significantly symptomatic lesions and is planned on a case-by-case basis.

Clinical scenario: a patient with a venous malformation

Presentation: A 27-year-old female teacher presented to her GP with a swelling over her lateral right thigh that had got progressively worse over the past 2 years and was now causing her pain, particularly on standing for long periods of time. She was otherwise fit and well.

Examination findings: She generally looked well. She pointed to an area supero-lateral to her right patella where there was mild swelling. There was no joint effusion or clinical findings attributable to any knee joint pathology. No tenderness or pulsatility was elicited. On standing, the swelling became more prominent and was slightly boggy on palpation.

Differential diagnosis: Vascular malformation, soft tissue tumour (much less likely given the above-mentioned history). Referral to vascular clinic or AVM specialist clinic.

Investigations: Duplex scan.

Results: Duplex scan demonstrated multiple dilated vascular channels with low flow on colour Doppler imaging in keeping with a vascular malformation. There were no atypical or solid features to suggest a more sinister cause that would be investigated with an MRI scan followed by referral to a sarcoma MDT.

Management: Compression hosiery, consideration for further imaging – MRI. Advised to use aspirin as required for any acute episodes of pain and avoid oral contraceptive pill.

Outcome: The patient gained some relief from wearing compression hosiery, but was still symptomatic so she was referred for MRI of the right thigh. This demonstrated serpiginous vascular channels subcutaneously in lateral aspect of the thigh. The patient underwent sclerotherapy by direct injection of sclerosant foam into the lesion, with subsequent reduction in symptoms. She returned for two further sessions of sclerotherapy with ongoing good clinical outcome and no complications.

Further reading

Dompartin A, Vikkula M, Boon LM. Venous malformation: update on aetiopathogenesis, diagnosis and management. *Phlebology* 2010; **25**:224–235.

Donnelly LF, Adams DM, Bisset GS. Vascular malformations and hemangiomas: a practical approach in a multidisciplinary clinic. *American Journal of Roentgenology*. 2000;**174**:597–608.

Jackson J. Vascular anomalies. In: Beard J.D. *et al.*, eds. *Vascular and endovascular surgery*, 5th edn, pp. 346–354. Elsevier, Saunders.

McCafferty IJ, Jones RG. Imaging and management of vascular malformations. *Clin Radiol* 2011;**66**:1208–1218.

CHAPTER 14

Secondary Prevention and Antiplatelet Therapy in Peripheral Arterial Disease

Richard Donnelly

Division of Medical Sciences & GEM, School of Medicine, University of Nottingham, UK

OVERVIEW

- Symptomatic PAD (peripheral arterial disease) is an important clinical indicator of high CV (cardiovascular) risk because atherosclerosis in the lower limbs is invariably associated with disease (which may be subclinical) in other vascular territories, especially the heart. More severe PAD [as reflected by a lower ABPI (ankle-brachial pressure index)] is associated with a higher mortality from CV disease

- Most of the major trials that have demonstrated the benefits of secondary prevention included subgroups of patients with symptomatic PAD. It is much less clear whether this evidence of benefit would also apply to patients with asymptomatic PAD identified by population screening of ABPI

- The mainstay of secondary prevention includes lifestyle measures (especially smoking cessation), BP (blood pressure)-lowering, lipid-lowering and antiplatelet drugs

- Antihypertensive therapy typically requires more than one drug to achieve BP goals and should ideally include an ACE (angiotensin-converting enzyme) inhibitor. Lipid-lowering therapy (ideally with a statin) should target LDL (low-density lipoprotein)- and non-HDL (high-density lipoprotein)-cholesterol reduction

- Antiplatelet therapy is indicated in patients with symptomatic PAD. In patients with very high CV risk, e.g. those undergoing revascularisation or with critical limb ischaemia, combination antiplatelet therapy may be required despite a higher risk of bleeding.

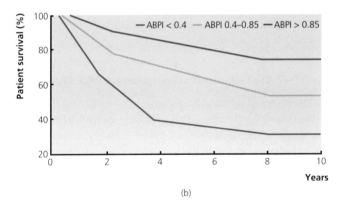

Figure 14.1 (a) Survival curves for patients with symptomatic and asymptomatic PAD, and those with severe symptoms (e.g. critical limb ischaemia), in a population cohort (data from Criqui *et al.*, 1992) and (b) survival among patients with PAD according to ankle-brachial pressure index (ABPI). ABPI is an independent predictor of mortality. Source: McKenna *et al.* (1991). Reproduced by permission of Elsevier.

Introduction

Patients with peripheral arterial disease (PAD), especially those with symptoms, have a 3- to 4-fold increased risk of cardiovascular (CV) mortality as a result of atherosclerosis in other vascular territories, particularly the coronary and cerebral circulations. Furthermore, in population studies, the severity of PAD as measured by the ankle-brachial pressure index (ABPI) correlates with reduced survival (Figure 14.1). Thus, symptomatic PAD is indicative of systemic vascular disease – it is as important a prognostic marker as stable angina or recent myocardial infarction (MI) – and therefore patients should be treated with lifestyle and drug interventions as part of secondary prevention to improve lower limb and CV outcomes.

Most trials of secondary prevention have included patients with known, symptomatic PAD (e.g. those with intermittent claudication or previous revascularisation), but whether treatment recommendations for secondary prevention would apply to asymptomatic patients with PAD, e.g. those identified by population screening of ABPI, is unclear. In observational studies, however, treatment with two or more preventative therapies [including aspirin, statin and/or

ABC of Arterial and Venous Disease, Third Edition.
Edited by Tim England and Akhtar Nasim.
© 2015 John Wiley & Sons, Ltd. Published 2015 by John Wiley & Sons, Ltd.

ACE (angiotensin-converting enzyme) inhibitor] was associated with a 65% reduced risk of all-cause mortality in individuals with PAD who had not previously had any symptoms of CV disease.

In surveys of routine clinical practice, a large proportion of patients with PAD fail to receive optimum secondary prevention (Box 14.1), in part because clinicians have misjudged the prognostic significance of lower limb symptoms. In the United States, it is estimated that 5m adults with PAD are not taking a statin and 4.4m are not receiving antiplatelet therapy.

Box 14.1 Major risk factors for progression of arterial disease and life-threatening CV complications of atherosclerosis.

- Age
- Known CV disease, including PAD
- Cigarette smoking
- High blood pressure
- Total and LDL-cholesterol
- Diabetes
- Atrial fibrillation*

*Atrial fibrillation is common in patients with PAD and associated with a higher risk of various unwanted outcomes, including thromboembolic limb ischaemia and stroke.

Lifestyle advice

Education and lifestyle changes should focus on smoking cessation, diet, weight management, moderation of alcohol consumption and regular physical activity (Box 14.2).

Box 14.2 Key components of lifestyle advice (NICE clinical guideline 172).

Smoking
- Encourage all people who smoke to stop and offer referral to a smoking cessation service.

Diet
- Advise a Mediterranean-style diet, e.g.:
  - more bread, vegetables, fruit and fish
  - less meat
  - replace butter and cheese with products based on plant oils
  - do not recommend routinely eating oily fish.

Weight control
- Provide patients who are overweight or obese with dietary advice and information to achieve and maintain a healthy weight (NICE guideline CG43).

Alcohol intake
- Weekly consumption should not exceed 21 units for men and 14 units for women.
- Avoid binge drinking (no more than three alcoholic drinks in 1–2 h).

Physical activity
- Advise people to be physically active for 20–30 min per day to the point of slight breathlessness.

- People who are not active to this level should gradually increase the duration and intensity of activity.

Fatty acid supplements
- According to NICE (CG 172), there is no basis for advising people to take omega-3 fatty acid capsules or omega-3 fatty acid supplemented foods (nor is there any evidence of harm from these products).

Smoking is strongly associated with PAD. Observational studies have shown that mortality and amputation rates are considerably higher, and revascularisation patency rates are much lower, among PAD patients who continue to smoke. In those who are motivated and supported, smoking cessation interventions, e.g. nicotine replacement therapy (NRT), alleviate short-term nicotine withdrawal symptoms and increase long-term quit rates by 2- to 3-fold. Bupropion and varenicline, a nicotine receptor partial agonist, are alternatives to NRT for managing the symptoms associated with abrupt smoking cessation. Varenicline achieves higher quit rates than NRT in randomised trials but is associated with a higher incidence of behavioural or mood changes such as agitation, depression and suicidal thoughts.

The CV benefits of smoking cessation accrue fairly quickly – e.g. up to 50% risk reduction within 1–2 years – whereas the excess cancer risks associated with smoking persist for much longer. Thus, smoking cessation services are very cost-effective for CV risk reduction.

Regular exercise (e.g. brisk 30-min walks three or four times per week) may improve walking distances in patients with PAD but exercise has other metabolic, haemodynamic and CV benefits. The best evidence of the benefits of exercise originates from randomised trials in the context of cardiac rehabilitation.

Lipid-lowering therapy

The Heart Protection study (HPS) demonstrated the benefits of statin therapy (simvastatin 40 mg) in patients with symptomatic PAD and a total-cholesterol level >3.5 mmol/L (Figure 14.2). American Heart Association guidelines (2013) have emphasised the wider CV benefits of cholesterol reduction (e.g. stroke prevention), the superiority and safety of statins over other lipid-lowering drugs, and highlighted the evidence that more intensive statin treatment is better than less intensive treatment to maximise CV risk reduction.

Although there is debate about whether statins have non-lipid-mediated (e.g. anti-inflammatory) effects that contribute to their mode of action, in a combined analysis of major statin trials, improvements in CV outcomes were in proportion to the reduction in LDL (low-density lipoprotein)-cholesterol. A subgroup analysis of the 4S study also showed that in patients with PAD statin therapy reduces the incidence of new or worsening claudication.

Target levels of total- and LDL-cholesterol of <4 and <2 mmol/L, respectively, should be used to titrate statin treatment in secondary prevention (Figure 14.3). Monitoring lipid levels is important

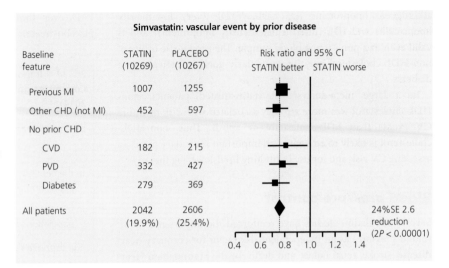

Figure 14.2 caption and table:

Baseline feature	STATIN (10269)	PLACEBO (10267)	Risk ratio and 95% CI STATIN better STATIN worse
Previous MI	1007	1255	
Other CHD (not MI)	452	597	
No prior CHD			
CVD	182	215	
PVD	332	427	
Diabetes	279	369	
All patients	2042 (19.9%)	2606 (25.4%)	24% SE 2.6 reduction (2P < 0.00001)

Simvastatin: vascular event by prior disease

Figure 14.2 The Heart Protection study was a large placebo-controlled trial of simvastatin 40 mg daily in a population of patients treated for primary and secondary prevention with average or low levels of cholesterol (>3.5 mmol/L). The subgroup with known peripheral vascular disease (PVD) at baseline achieved as much benefit from statin therapy as those with prior myocardial infarction. Source: Heart Protection Study Collaborative Group (2002). Reproduced by permission of Elsevier.

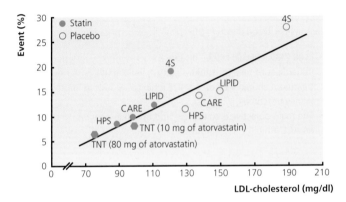

Figure 14.3 This analysis plots the achieved cholesterol level in both the placebo-treated and statin-treated groups in each of the major statin trials against the observed CV event rates, for example, in the 4S, CARE and Heart Protection studies (HPS). It reinforces the notion that lower is better. Data from La Rosa *et al.* (2005).

because fewer than half of the patients will achieve these targets using simvastatin 40 mg daily. Substitution of a more potent statin (e.g. atorvastatin or rosuvastatin), up-titration to simvastatin 80 mg daily or use of additional lipid-lowering treatments, e.g. ezetimibe, may be required in order to achieve optimum LDL-cholesterol reduction. Musculoskeletal aches and pains, and changes in liver function, are the commonest side effects of statin treatment.

Although LDL-cholesterol is the primary measurement used for initiating and titrating lipid-lowering therapy, there is emerging evidence that LDL-cholesterol may not be the best lipid marker to predict CV risk or the anti-atherosclerotic effect of statin therapy. Alternative measurements, in particular, apolipoprotein B (apo-B, which is not routinely measured in most clinical laboratories) and non-HDL (high-density lipoprotein)-cholesterol, have been shown in population studies to be superior to LDL-cholesterol in assessing CV risk (Figure 14.4). Non-HDL-cholesterol is easily calculated by the clinician: total-cholesterol level minus the HDL-cholesterol level. It reflects the sum of serum cholesterol carried by all the

What is Non-HDL-C?

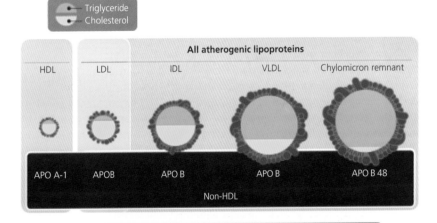

Figure 14.4 Non-HDL-cholesterol is emerging as an important secondary lipid target for use in assessing CV risk and for titration of lipid-lowering therapy. It may correlate more closely with future CV risk.

atherogenic lipoproteins [i.e. LDL, VLDL (very low-density lipoprotein) and IDL (intermediate-density lipoprotein)] and is valid even in a non-fasting blood sample. The prognostic utility of non-HDL-cholesterol may be particularly good in patients with diabetes.

In a large meta-analysis of statin-treated patients, non-HDL-cholesterol was more strongly associated with risk of future CV events than LDL-cholesterol or apo-B. Thus, non-HDL-cholesterol is likely to emerge as an important secondary target in assessing CV risk and for use in titrating lipid-lowering therapy.

Blood pressure control

Several population studies have reinforced the importance of BP (blood pressure) as an independent risk factor for coronary heart disease, stroke, renal failure and death. In the Framingham Heart study, the risk of intermittent claudication was 2.5- to 4-fold higher among hypertensive patients compared with controls. Furthermore, small differences in BP, maintained over several years, translate into large differences in CV outcomes. Therefore, detecting and treating high BP remains one of the most cost-effective public health interventions to reduce the population incidence of CV disease. Placebo-adjusted treatment effects of around 10/5 mmHg result in 30–40% relative risk reductions in stroke and 15–20% reductions in major coronary disease events.

Several studies have shown that CV end-organ damage associated with hypertension is more strongly correlated with 24-h ambulatory blood pressure (ABP) than with clinic or casual BP measurements (Box 14.3). ABP monitoring requires specialised, validated machines and careful quality control measures. Interpretation of the ABP profile typically includes measurements of mean daytime, night-time (asleep) and 24-h BP. Normal BP values for adults are <135/85 mmHg for daytime, <120/75 mmHg for night-time and <130/80 mmHg for 24-h BP.

Box 14.3 Clinical uses of 24-h ambulatory BP monitoring

- To exclude 'white coat' hypertension
- To investigate apparent 'drug-resistant' hypertension
- Investigation of symptomatic hypotension, e.g. in the elderly
- To assess adequacy of BP control in patients at high CV risk

---

Recent guidelines from the Eighth Joint National Committee (JNC-8) in the United States have clarified recommendations with respect to thresholds for BP intervention and target levels of BP control among those on treatment (Box 14.4).

In the general (non-Black) population, including those with diabetes, initial antihypertensive treatment should include a thiazide-like diuretic, ACE inhibitor or calcium channel blocker (CCB) (Figure 14.5). Whether ACE inhibitors confer additional CV benefits that are independent of BP reduction is still uncertain, but these drugs are well established in the management of patients with heart failure, chronic kidney disease and those with diabetic nephropathy. In the HOPE trial, ACE inhibitor treatment reduced the risk of major CV events by 25% in patients with symptomatic

PAD, even though the difference in BP between Ramipril and placebo-treated patients was relatively small (3/2 mmHg).

Box 14.4 Important recommendations from the Joint National Committee guidelines (JNC-8) on hypertension (published 2014).

	Initiate BP-lowering treatment	Goal
In the general population ≥60 years:	SBP ≥150 or DBP ≥90 mmHg	<150/90
In the general population <60 years:	SBP ≥140 or DBP ≥90 mmHg	<140/90
In patients with CKD:	SBP ≥140 or DBP ≥90 mmHg	<140/90
In patients with diabetes:	SBP ≥140 or DBP ≥90 mmHg	<140/90

SBP, systolic blood pressure; DBP, diastolic blood pressure.

- In all CKD (chronic kidney disease) patients with hypertension (regardless of race or diabetes status), initial antihypertensive treatment should include an ACE inhibitor or ARB to improve kidney outcomes.
- The main objective is to achieve and maintain goal BP. Do not use an ACE inhibitor and ARB together.

Angiotensin receptor antagonists (ARAs) are generally reserved for patients who are intolerant of ACE inhibitors (usually because of a dry cough).

Three-quarters of patients will require combination BP-lowering therapy (25% will need triple therapy) and approximately 10% will have resistant hypertension (defined as inadequate BP control despite treatment with 3–4 drugs). Difficult-to-treat systolic hypertension due to arterial stiffness and atheromatous reno-vascular disease are more common in patients with PAD. Renal (sympathetic) denervation has been developed for patients with drug-resistant hypertension. A catheter placed sequentially in each of the renal arteries delivers high-frequency radio waves to disrupt perivascular sympathetic nerves. Although initial studies reported significant and sustained BP reductions, the role of this technique has yet to be established in randomised trials.

Antiplatelet therapy

Atherosclerosis produces an inherently thrombogenic inner surface on affected blood vessels. In addition, ulceration and rupture of atherosclerotic plaques often triggers platelet activation and aggregation followed by local thrombus formation and complete vessel occlusion. This cascade of events may then result in life-threatening, unstable disease causing an acute coronary syndrome, acute stroke or acute limb ischaemia. Thus, antiplatelet therapy has an important role in secondary prevention.

The platelet surface membrane is rich in receptors and adhesion proteins that co-ordinate interactions among the platelet, other

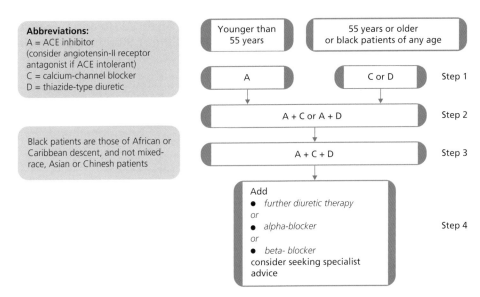

Figure 14.5 The British Hypertension Society guidelines for drug selection and combination therapy in hypertension. Note that beta-blockers are no longer used in steps 1–3. ARBs are used when an ACE inhibitor is not tolerated. If BP control is inadequate despite maximum doses of A + C + D, options include adding an alpha-adrenoceptor antagonist (e.g. doxazosin), spironolactone, moxonidine or a beta-blocker.

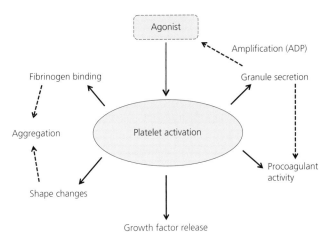

Figure 14.6 Binding of various agonists to the platelet (e.g. ADP, collagen and thromboxane A_2) leads to a cascade reaction of amplification and platelet aggregation. This in turn binds fibrinogen and promotes thrombus formation, e.g. on the surface of a ruptured atheromatous plaque.

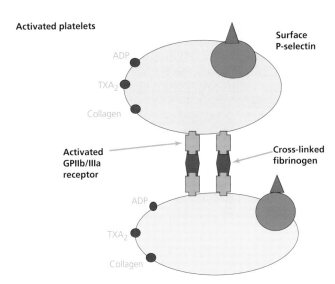

Figure 14.7 Thromboxane, ADP and collagen bind to receptors on the platelet surface. Activation of the platelet leads to shape change, aggregation and activation of the glycoprotein IIb/IIIa receptor. Fibrinogen cross-linking promotes platelet aggregation and thrombus formation.

platelets, components of the blood and the vessel wall. Production of thromboxane $A_2 (TXA_2)$ in response to various stimuli has an important role in the amplification of platelet activation and vaso-constriction. Various agonists trigger platelet activation by binding to specific receptors (e.g. TXA_2, collagen and ADP receptors) which in turn activate the glycoprotein IIb/IIIa (GP IIb/IIIa) receptor and cause platelet cross-linking via binding fibrinogen (Figures 14.6 and 14.7).

$P2Y_{12}$ is the predominant receptor involved in ADP-stimulated platelet activation of the GP IIb/IIIa receptor. Binding of ADP to $P2Y_{12}$ stimulates activation of the GP IIb/IIIa receptor resulting in platelet degranulation, thromboxane production and prolonged aggregation.

A number of antiplatelet drugs are available that act on different receptors and pathways involved in platelet-mediated thrombogenesis (Box 14.5). Aspirin acts by irreversibly acetylating cyclooxygenase-1 and -2 (COX-1 and COX-2), thereby inhibiting formation of TXA_2 and the vasodilator prostacyclin. Endothelial cells can regenerate COX but platelets are anucleate and cannot regenerate the enzyme. Thus, the inhibitory effect of aspirin on endothelial prostacyclin is only transient, whereas its effect on platelets is permanent.

The thienopyridines, e.g. clopidogrel and prasugrel, bind irreversibly to the platelet ADP ($P2Y_{12}$ subtype) receptor. Clopidogrel and prasugrel are pro-drugs, activated in the liver, and have more powerful antiplatelet effects than aspirin. The newer drugs, cangrelor and ticagrelor, are direct-acting reversible $P2Y_{12}$ inhibitors.

Box 14.5 **Antiplatelet drugs**

Mode of action	Antiplatelet drugs
Cyclooxygenase inhibitors	Aspirin, ibuprofen, sulphinpyrazone
ADP ($P2Y_{12}$) receptor blockers	Clopidogrel, ticagrelor, prasugrel
Glycoprotein IIb/IIIa inhibitors	Tirofiban, eptifibatide, abciximab
Phosphodiesterase inhibitors	Dipyridamole, cilostazol
Thromboxane synthase inhibitors	Picotamide

The glycoprotein IIb/IIIa inhibitors tend to be used for short term as peri-procedural adjuncts to aspirin and heparin in patients with acute coronary syndromes undergoing a percutaneous coronary intervention.

Aspirin, in daily doses of 75–325 mg (reflecting heterogeneity of doses in clinical trials), is recommended to reduce the risk of MI, stroke or vascular death in patients with PAD, including those with claudication, critical limb ischaemia or prior lower limb revascularisation. The POPADAD (prevention of progression of arterial disease and diabetes) study was placebo-controlled and found no benefit of low dose aspirin in patients with diabetes and asymptomatic PAD. An updated meta-analysis in 2009 that included both symptomatic and asymptomatic PAD patients demonstrated a 34% risk reduction in nonfatal stroke among patients treated with aspirin but the overall reduction in CV events was non-significant. The strongest evidence of benefit is in those patients with lower limb symptoms.

On the basis of the CHARISMA (Clopidogrel for High Atherothrombotic Risk and Ischemic Stabilization, Management, and Avoidance) trial, combination therapy with aspirin + clopidogrel should be considered for those PAD patients who are considered to be at especially high risk of CV disease and who are not at increased risk of bleeding. This might include patients with critical limb ischaemia or those undergoing a revascularisation procedure (e.g. stenting). In acute coronary syndrome patients, aspirin + clopidogrel or ticagrelor is recommended for up to 12 months (NICE guidance).

The WAVE trial provided evidence against the use of oral anticoagulants in addition to antiplatelet therapy among patients with PAD.

Glycaemic control

Micro- and macrovascular disease in the lower limbs are major contributors to diabetes-related foot complications, e.g. ulceration and amputations. Atherosclerosis in patients with diabetes tends to be more diffuse, distal and calcified and therefore less amenable to revascularisation and stenting. Glycaemic control, as measured by glycosylated haemoglobin (HbA1c), is most closely associated with microvascular complications, e.g. diabetic retinopathy and nephropathy. In both type 1 and type 2 diabetes, a so-called legacy effect has been observed, whereby reductions in HbA1c in the first few years after diagnosis result in CV benefits that become evident 10–20 years later. Thus, guidelines tend to favour tighter glycaemic control (e.g. HbA1c <6.5%) in the first few years (i.e. steps 1 and 2 in the NICE guideline for type 2 diabetes) and less tight control

Glycated Hb and CV outcomes: NZ Cohort Study (48,000 patients T2D)

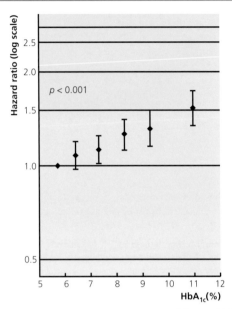

Diabet Med 2008; 25:1295

Figure 14.8 An observational cohort study from New Zealand in 48 000 patients showing the linear relationship between HbA1c and CV diseases. Source: Elley *et al.* (2008). Reproduced with permission from John Wiley and Sons.

(e.g. HbA1c <7.5%) in patients with longer duration disease where the risk–benefit balance may be influenced by hypoglycaemic risk and diminished hypoglycaemic awareness.

There is a linear relationship between HbA1c and CV outcomes, even in the non-diabetic range (Figure 14.8), but intervention trials in type 2 diabetes have shown that BP and lipid-lowering strategies are more effective than lowering HbA1c in preventing CV events (Figure 14.9).

Intensive glucose-lowering: absolute number of Events Prevented per 1000 patient-yrs of treatment*

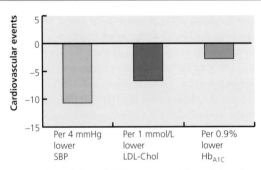

*Data from cholesterol & BP-treatment trialists collaboration.

Preiss D, et al. Br. Med. J 2011 ; 343: d4243

Figure 14.9 Absolute number of CV events prevented per 1000 patient – years of treatment showing the comparative effectiveness of intensive BP, glucose and lipid lowering. Data from Preiss 2011.

Conclusions

Symptomatic PAD is an important prognostic indicator of high CV risk because atherosclerosis in the lower limbs is invariably associated with disease in other vascular territories, especially the heart. In order to reduce the risk of limb- or life-threatening complications, patients with PAD should receive secondary prevention with evidence-based, disease-modifying drugs that have been shown to reduce CV risk. This includes BP- and lipid-lowering treatment, lifestyle modification and antiplatelet therapy. Regular surveillance and adjustment of treatment is needed to ensure maximal CV risk reduction.

Further reading

Alnaeb ME, Alobaid N, Seifalian AM, *et al*. Statins and peripheral arterial disease: potential mechanisms and clinical benefits. *Ann Vasc Surg* 2006;**20**:696–705.

American College of Cardiology Foundation, American Heart Association Task Force, Society for Cardiovascular Angiography and Interventions, Rooke TW, *et al*. 2011 ACCF/AHA focused update of the guideline for the management of patients with peripheral artery disease. *Circulation* 2011;**124**:2020–2045.

Anand S, Yusuf S, Xie C, *et al*. Oral anticoagulant and antiplatelet therapy and peripheral arterial disease. *N Engl J Med* 2007;**357**:217–227.

Antiplatelet Trialists Collaboration. Collaborative overview of randomised trials of antiplatelet therapy, I: prevention of death, myocardial infarction and stroke by prolonged antiplatelet therapy in various categories of patients. *BMJ* 1994;**308**:81–106.

Berger JS, Krantz MJ, Kittelson JM, *et al*. Aspirin for the prevention of cardiovascular events in patients with peripheral arterial disease: a meta-analysis of randomised trials. *JAMA* 2009;**301**:1909–1919.

Boekholdt SM, Arsenault BJ, Mora S, *et al*. Association of LDL cholesterol, Non-HDL-cholesterol, and apolipoprotein B levels with risk of cardiovascular events among patients treated with statins: a meta-analysis. *JAMA* 2012;**307**:1302–1309.

Cacoub PP, Bhatt DL, Steg PG, *et al*. Patients with peripheral arterial disease in the CHARISMA trial. *Eur Heart J* 2009;**30**:192–201.

Criqui MH, Langer RD, Fronek A, *et al*. Mortality over a period of 10 years in patients with peripheral arterial disease. *N Engl J Med* 1992;**326**:381–386.

Dagher NN and Modrall JG. Pharmacotherapy before and after revascularization: anticoagulation, antiplatelet agents, and statins. *Semin Vasc Surg* 2007;**20**:10–14.

Elley CR, Kenealy T, Robinson E and Drury PL. Glycated haemoglobin and cardiovascular outcomes in people with type 2 diabetes: a large prospective cohort study. *Diabet Med* 2008;**25**(11):1295–1301.

Heart Protection Study Collaborative Group. MRC/BHF Heart Protection Study of cholesterol lowering with simvastatin in 20,536 high risk individuals: a randomized placebo controlled trail. *Lancet* 2002;**360**:7–22.

Heart Protection Study Collaborative Group. Randomised trial of the effects of cholesterol-lowering with simvastatin on peripheral vascular and other major vascular outcomes in 20,536 people with peripheral arterial disease and other high-risk conditions. *J Vasc Surg* 2007;**45**:645–654.

James PA, Oparil S, Carter BL, *et al*. Evidence-based guideline for the management of high BP in adults: report from the panel members appointed to the Eighth Joint National Committee (JNC-8). *JAMA* 2014. doi:10.1001/jama.2013.284427.

Jones K, Saxon L, Cunningham W and Adams P. Secondary prevention for patients after a myocardial infarction: summary of updated NICE guidance. *BMJ* 2013;**347**:f6544. doi:10.1136/bmj.f6544 (published November 13th 2013).

LaRosa JC, Grundy SM, Walters DD, *et al*. Intensive lipid lowering with atorvastatin in patients with stable coronary heart disease. *N Engl J Med* 2005;**352**:1425–1435.

McKenna M, Wolfson S and Kuller L. The ratio of ankle and arm arterial pressure as an independent predictor of mortality. *Atherosclerosis* 1991;**87**:119–128.

Mehler PS, Coll JR, Estacio R, *et al*. Intensive blood pressure control reduces the risk of cardiovascular events in patients with peripheral arterial disease and type 2 diabetes. *Circulation* 2003a;**107**:753–756.

Mehler PS, Coll JR, Estacio R, *et al*. Intensive blood pressure control reduces the risk of cardiovascular events in patients with peripheral arterial disease and type 2 diabetes. *Circulation* 2003b;**107**:753–756.

National Institute for Health and Care Excellence. Secondary prevention in primary and secondary care for patients following a myocardial infarction. (Clinical guideline 172), 2013. www.nice.org.uk/CG172.

Pande RL, Perlstein TS, Beckman JA and Craeger MA. Secondary prevention and mortality in peripheral artery disease. National health and nutrition examination study, 1999 to 2004. *Circulation* 2011;**124**:17–23.

Paraskevas KI, Kotsikoris I, Koupidis SA, *et al*. Ankle-brachial index: a marker of both peripheral arterial disease and systemic atherosclerosis as well as a predictor of vascular events. *Angiology* 2010;**61**:521–523.

Preiss D. Intensive glucose lowering treatment in type 2 diabetes *BMJ* 2011; **343** d4243

Sobel M and Verhaeghe R. American College of Chest Physicians. Antithrombotic therapy for peripheral artery occlusive disease: American College of Chest Physicians evidence-based clinical practice guidelines (8th edition). *Chest* 2008;**133**:815S–843S.

Stone NJU, Robinson J, Lichtenstein AH, *et al*. ACC/AHA guideline on the treatment of blood cholesterol to reduce atherosclerotic cardiovascular risk in adults: a report of the American College of cardiology/American Heart Association Task Force on Practice Guidelines. *J Am Coll Cardiol* 2013. doi:10.1016/j.jacc.2013.11.002.

Tendera M, Aboyans V, *et al*. ESC Guidelines on the diagnosis and treatment of peripheral artery diseases: document covering atherosclerotic disease of extracranial carotid and vertebral, mesenteric, renal, upper and lower extremity arteries: the task force on the diagnosis and treatment of peripheral artery diseases of the European Society of Cardiology (ESC). *Eur Heart J* 2011;**32**:2851–2906.

CHAPTER 15

Anticoagulants in Venous and Arterial Disease

Sue Pavord and Amy Webster

Department of Haematology, University Hospital of Leicester NHS Trust, UK

OVERVIEW

- Anticoagulation is the mainstay of treatment for venous thromboembolic disease and prevention of stroke and systemic embolism in patients with atrial fibrillation (AF)
- Heparin and vitamin K antagonists have been the only available anticoagulants for several decades but the recent introduction of novel orally active anticoagulants is changing the way that many of these patients are managed
- The duration of anticoagulation after acute venous thromboembolism (VTE) needs to be assessed on an individual basis
- The risk of VTE in medical and surgical patients has been highlighted in recent years and much attention has been given to risk assessment and thrombosis prevention measures.

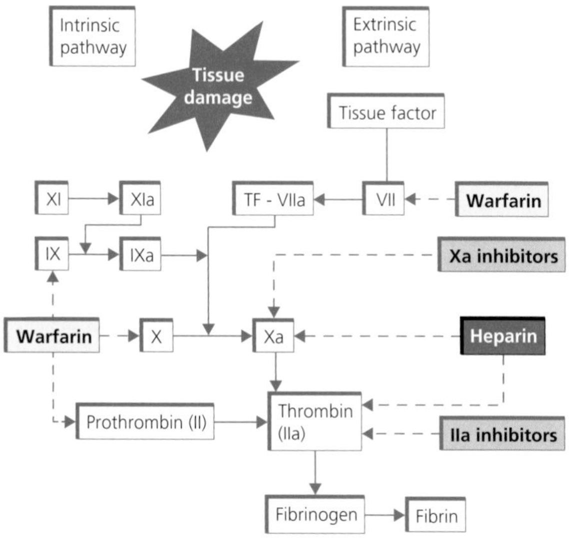

Figure 15.1 Coagulation system and sites of inhibition by different anticoagulants.

Heparin

Heparins are naturally occurring sulphated glycosaminoglycans isolated from animal tissue, most commonly porcine intestine. They indirectly inhibit blood coagulation, through their effect on antithrombin. A specific five-sugar (pentasaccharide) sequence of the heparin molecule binds with high affinity to antithrombin, inducing conformational change and enhancing its inhibitory activity by some 2000-fold. The main effect is on thrombin and factor Xa, key factors in the coagulation cascade and development of the fibrin clot (Figure 15.1).

Heparin is widely used for therapeutic and prophylactic anticoagulation. It has a rapid onset of action and short half-life but can only be administered parenterally due to its rapid destruction by gut enzymes.

Unfractionated heparin (UFH)

The mean molecular weight of UFH (unfractionated heparin) is 15 000 Da, which allows it to bind to both antithrombin and thrombin, giving both anti-IIa and anti-Xa activity in roughly equal measure. It is given intravenously and requires a loading dose before continuous infusion. Doses are adjusted according to the activated partial thromboplastin time (APTT), which should be measured every 6 h until stable. The therapeutic APTT range depends on the sensitivity of the reagent used and needs to be determined locally. The required doses to achieve therapeutic anticoagulation can be variable due to the non-specific binding to plasma proteins.

The use of UFH in first-line treatment for VTE (venous thromboembolism) has largely been superseded by low molecular weight heparin (LMWH) and oral direct inhibitors (NOACS), although UFH is still useful for patients with renal impairment.

Low molecular weight heparin (LMWH)

LMWHs are produced by chemical or enzymatic cleavage of UFH. The action of LMWH is primarily on anti-Xa, as the smaller molecular size (3000–5000 Da) renders it unable to form a tertiary ternary heparin–thrombin–antithrombin complex required for the inactivation of thrombin (Figure 15.2).

LMWH is given by subcutaneous injection and has more predictable pharmacokinetics, largely because of the lack of non-specific plasma protein binding. Dosing is weight dependent, and maybe once or twice daily, dependent on the preparation. Excretion is primarily renal and dosing adjustments may be required in renal impairment. Monitoring is not routinely required,

ABC of Arterial and Venous Disease, Third Edition.
Edited by Tim England and Akhtar Nasim.
© 2015 John Wiley & Sons, Ltd. Published 2015 by John Wiley & Sons, Ltd.

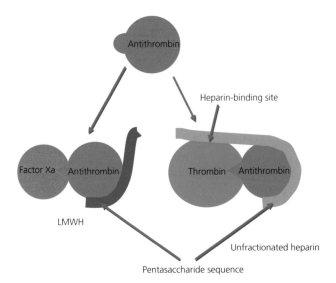

Figure 15.2 Heparin binding to antithrombin. Only heparins of more than 18 saccharide units can complex antithrombin to thrombin.

Table 15.1 Comparison of unfractionated and low molecular weight heparins.

Unfractionated heparin	Low molecular weight heparin
Increased half-life with increased concentration of drug (range 30 min to 4 h)	Stable half-life, ~4 h, and more predictable dose response
Non-specific protein binding	Reduced non-specific binding
<50% bioavailability subcutaneously (at low dosage)	>90% bioavailability subcutaneously
Monitoring required with APTT	No monitoring required (anti-Xa if occasionally needed)
Risk of heparin-induced thrombocytopenia	Lower risk of heparin-induced thrombocytopenia
Hepatic and renal elimination	Renal elimination
Risk of osteoporosis with prolonged therapy	Lower risk of osteoporosis

but in cases of renal failure or extremes of weight, measurement of anti-Xa activity can be helpful. LMWH has been shown to be as effective as UFH in the treatment of VTE and allows for outpatient management in suitable patients. Other advantages of LMWH are shown in Table 15.1.

Fondaparinux

Fondaparinux is a synthetic pentasaccharide, chemically related to the antithrombin-binding site of heparin. Like heparin, it has to be administered parenterally and is used for the prevention and treatment of VTE.

Vitamin K antagonists

Vitamin K is required as a cofactor for the conversion of glutamic acid to γ-carboxyglutamic acid in the synthesis of coagulation factors II, VII, IX and X (Figure 15.3) and the natural anticoagulants, proteins S and C. Vitamin K antagonists, of which warfarin is most commonly used, competitively inhibit this process. The peak pharmacological effect is at approximately 48 h post dose because

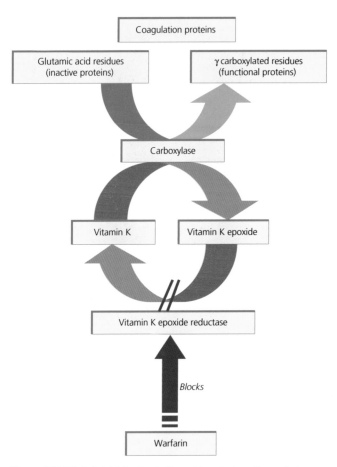

Figure 15.3 Warfarin inhibits vitamin K epoxide reductase, thus reducing functional coagulation protein synthesis.

of the time taken for degradation of existing clotting factors. Furthermore, the initial period can be associated with transient hypercoagulability due to the reduction in the natural anticoagulant proteins C and S, which have shorter half-lives than the procoagulant factors II, IX and X. This occurs despite a prolonged INR (international normalised ratio), which is largely determined by the fall in FVII. Therefore, on starting warfarin for treatment of VTE, concomitant LMWH should be given for at least 5 days.

Warfarin is orally bioavailable and rapidly absorbed in the gastrointestinal tract. It is metabolised by the hepatic cytochrome P450 system and is highly plasma protein bound, causing many pharmacological interactions and variation in half-life between patients. It, therefore, requires close monitoring and often minor dose changes to ensure stable anticoagulation. Factors influencing warfarin control are outlined in Box 15.1.

Box 15.1 **Factors influencing stability of warfarin control**

Drugs and other factors influencing anticoagulation with warfarin
- Acquired factors
  - Acute illness
  - Impaired liver function
  - Renal failure
  - Excess alcohol
  - Diet poor in vitamin K
- Inherited factors

- Increasing sensitivity – CYP2C9 mutation
- Causing resistance – VKORC1 mutation
- Drugs enhancing anticoagulation
  - Reduced protein binding: aspirin, chlorpromazine, sulphonamides
  - Inhibition of warfarin metabolism: cimetidine, allopurinol, tricyclic antidepressants, metronidazole, erythromycin, sodium valproate
  - Reduced vitamin absorption: antibiotics, laxatives
  - Decreased clotting factor synthesis: cephalosporins, phenytoin
- Drugs reducing anticoagulation
  - Increased metabolism of warfarin: barbiturates, rifampicin, carbamazepine
  - Increased clotting factor synthesis: oral contraceptives

Table 15.2 Risk of bleeding according to level of INR.

INR	Relative bleeding risk
2.0–2.9	4.8
3–4.4	9.5
4.5–6.9	40.5
≥7	200

Source: Palareti et al. (1996). Reproduced by permission of Elsevier.

Warfarin is monitored using the prothrombin time (PT), which is expressed as the ratio of the PT of the patient to that of a pool of healthy donors. PT measurements have been standardised internationally by the use of an assigned international sensitivity index (ISI) to each thromboplastin reagent, which compares the reagent to a world standard. INR is then calculated as follows:

$$INR = (PT\ ratio)^{ISI}.$$

For most indications, including treatment of VTE, the target INR is 2.5 (range 2–3). If VTE recurs despite the INR being in the therapeutic range, the target should be increased to 3.5. Because the therapeutic range is narrow, there is a significant risk of over-anticoagulation and bleeding episodes are not infrequent. Table 15.2 indicates the increased risk of bleeding associated with high INRs.

Novel oral anticoagulants

Factor Xa inhibitors

Factor Xa inhibitors, such as rivaroxaban and apixaban, act by direct and selective inhibition of factor Xa (Figure 15.1). They are licensed for prevention of VTE following hip and knee arthroplasty and for stroke prevention in non-valvular atrial fibrillation (AF). Rivaroxaban is also licensed for treatment of acute VTE, with a recommended dose of 15 mg twice daily for the initial 3 weeks followed by 20 mg daily for completion of treatment. The majority of the drug undergoes hepatic metabolism and rivaroxaban is therefore contraindicated in moderate to severe hepatic dysfunction. Apixaban is likely to gain its licence in the near future, as data from

a large randomised controlled study have confirmed non-inferiority to conventional therapy in treatment of acute VTE. Both provide a predictable anticoagulant effect, obviating the need for monitoring. Owing to significant renal clearance, they are contraindicated in patients with a creatinine clearance <15 ml/min.

Direct thrombin inhibitors

Dabigatran etexilate is a pro-drug that is converted to its active form, dabigatran, after oral administration. It acts by competitive and reversible inhibition of thrombin, preventing the conversion of fibrinogen to fibrin (Figure 15.1). Elimination is primarily renal and dose adjustments should be made in renal impairment. Currently, it is licensed for VTE prevention following hip or knee replacement surgery and for stroke prevention in non-valvular AF. A large randomised controlled study (RE-COVER) showed that it was as effective as warfarin, with a similar bleeding profile, in the treatment of acute VTE.

Anticoagulation for acute venous disease

Anticoagulation for the treatment of PE (pulmonary embolism) and DVT (deep vein thrombosis) is the same and has two roles: initially preventing extension and propagation of thrombosis and thereafter preventing a recurrent event. The 2012 NICE guidelines recommend LMWH or fondaparinux as first-line agents, with UFH as an alternative in patients with renal impairment (eGFR < 30 ml/min), significant bleeding risk or in patients with PEs who are haemodynamically unstable and may require thrombolytic therapy. Vitamin K antagonists should be started simultaneously and both continued until the INR is >2 for at least 24 h. Subsequent guidelines also offer the oral direct inhibitors (NOACs) as an alternative, based on the data in prospective randomised controlled trials.

Inferior vena cava (IVC) filters are only recommended as a temporary option in those patients who have a contraindication to anticoagulation, such as active bleeding, and, if fitted, these should be removed when patients are eligible to start treatment (Figure 15.4).

Duration of anticoagulation

Proximal DVT (popliteal vein and above) and PE require at least 3 months of therapeutic anticoagulation. The duration of required anticoagulation thereafter is dependent on a number of factors (Box 15.2) but most importantly, the circumstances around the thrombotic event and the presence or absence of any provoking transient risk factors. For example, a patient with below-knee DVT following surgery is likely to need only 6 weeks of anticoagulation compared to an individual with spontaneous PE who would be considered for lifelong treatment. Where there is a clear provoking factor, such as surgery, or a transient risk factor that has resolved, such as pregnancy or the combined contraceptive pill, longer term anticoagulation is not usually recommended.

Unprovoked proximal VTE or PE is associated with a significant risk of recurrence of >9%. The decision to continue long-term anticoagulation needs to be balanced against the bleeding risks of

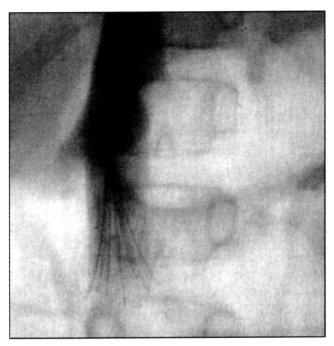

Figure 15.4 Vena cavagram showing umbrella delivery device for filter inserted into the inferior vena cava through the jugular vein. *Source*: Turpie *et al.* (2002). Reproduced by permission of BMJ Publishing Group Ltd.

the patient and reviewed periodically. Testing for heritable thrombophilia does not appear to predict the risk of recurrence and is not routinely recommended. Metaanalysis of clinical trials involving 1800 patients with unprovoked VTE enabled the development of a prediction score for VTE recurrence – $D_2A_1S_1H_{-2}$: 2 points for elevated D Dimers, 1 point for each of age over 50 years and male gender and minus 2 points for hormone therapy. A cumulative score of 2 or more was associated with an annual recurrence risk of 6.4% or more and felt to justify the continuation of anticoagulation if bleeding risk is acceptable.

Special circumstances

Pregnancy

Pregnancy and the postpartum period are associated with a 10–25-fold increased relative risk of VTE respectively, due to the natural increase in hypercoagulability as pregnancy advances.

Women with congenital or acquired thrombotic risk factors may require thromboprophylaxis in the antenatal period and for up to 6 weeks post partum to reduce their risk of a VTE. Diagnosis of a suspected VTE is more difficult in pregnancy, due to the high frequency of symptoms and signs that mimic DVT or PE and potential risks of lung scans for mother and baby.

Warfarin is teratogenic after 6 weeks of gestation and increases the risk of neonatal intracranial haemorrhage during delivery. Its use is therefore contraindicated and treatment of pregnancy-associated VTE is with therapeutic dose LMWH. Dose adjustment and anti-Xa levels may be required to ensure adequate anticoagulation. In the post partum period, LMWH can be substituted with warfarin for the remainder of the anticoagulation course. Both are safe to use during breast feeding.

Cancer

The risk of VTE is increased in patients with cancer and is associated with significant morbidity and mortality. Ten percent of the patients with idiopathic VTE are diagnosed with cancer in the next 2 years. Current NICE guidelines recommend treatment with LMWH, which confers a survival advantage over warfarin in this patient group and avoids the problems with warfarin in patients with heightened bleeding risks, multiple interventions and hepatic metastases. Treatment is required for at least 6 months, although the dose can be reduced after the first month if symptoms have resolved. At the end of the course, patients should be reassessed for ongoing thrombotic risk and may require continued prophylaxis.

Surgery

Surgery increases the risk of VTE through changes to the coagulation system, immobility and damage to the vessel walls. For patients on treatment for VTE, surgery should be postponed if possible. Otherwise, warfarin can be bridged with LMWH to provide stable anticoagulation with ease of interruption and minimise bleeding and thrombotic risks. Patients on oral direct inhibitors (NOACs, novel oral anticoagulants) should stop their anticoagulation 1–4 days before surgery, depending on renal function. If surgery is required within 1 week of thrombosis, a temporary IVC filter may be required.

Prevention of venous thromboembolism

Prevention of VTE should always be addressed in circumstances of known risk, such as pregnancy, surgery or hospital admission. Patient factors and the risks of surgery are assessed in determining the need for LMWH thromboprophylaxis and/or mechanical compression devices. All should receive written information and guidance on general measures such as hydration and feet and ankle exercises. Thromboprophylaxis is usually with LMWH. Guidelines produced by NICE and the Royal College of Obstetricians and Gynaecologists are helpful in outlining VTE prevention. In all cases, the risk of thrombosis should be balanced against the risk of bleeding.

Table 15.3 The CHADS-VASc scoring system for stroke risk factors in patients with AF.

	Risk factor	Score
C	Congestive heart failure/LV dysfunction	1
H	Hypertension	1
A2	Age ≥75 years	2
D	Diabetes mellitus	1
S2	Stroke/TIA/TE	2
V	Vascular disease (prior myocardial infarction, peripheral artery disease or aortic plaque)	1
A	Age 65–74 years	1
Sc	Sex category (i.e. female gender)	1
	Maximum score	9

Prevention of stroke in people with atrial fibrillation (AF)

Cardioembolism secondary to AF accounts for 30% of the ischaemic strokes. The embolic nature confers a significantly higher morbidity and mortality than those with strokes due to small vessel disease. The risk of stroke in patients with AF increases with the prevalence of other factors and can be assessed with the CHADS2 or CHADS2-VASc scoring system (Table 15.3). This needs to be offset against the risk of bleeding when considering use of anticoagulation, although the devastating consequences of stroke normally outweigh concerns about bleeding risk.

It has long been established that warfarin provides better stroke prevention therapy than aspirin, with two-thirds relative risk reduction. The bleeding risk of aspirin outweighs its efficacy in preventing cardioembolic stroke and there is no place for it, even in patients who are unable to take anticoagulants.

The oral direct inhibitors, rivaroxaban, apixaban and dabigatran, are licensed for stroke prevention in AF, having shown non-inferiority or superiority to warfarin in large randomised controlled trials. They provide stable, dose-dependent anticoagulation, without increased bleeding risk and the lack of required monitoring makes them an attractive option for many patients. They are not currently licensed for AF in association with heart valve disease. Figure 15.5 shows the guideline for management of patients with AF, produced by the European Society of Cardiology.

Complications of anticoagulation

Allergy
Delayed-type hypersensitivity reactions to LMWHs present as an itching or burning sensation at injection sites, associated with erythematous and sometimes excematous plaques, usually starting 1–2 weeks after the injection. Other LMWHs can be tried but often the reaction recurs and alternatives such as fondaparinux may be needed. Intravenous heparin is often tolerated and provocation testing is helpful to confirm this for future use.

Heparin-induced thrombocytopenia (HIT)
This rare immunological reaction is primarily seen with the use of UFH, due to its ability to activate platelets and release platelet

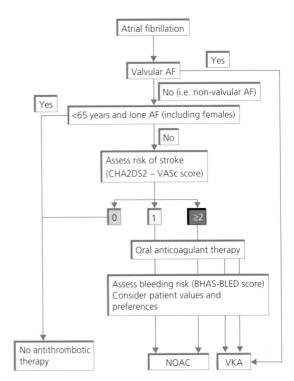

Figure 15.5 Algorithm of proposed management of patients with AF (data from the European Society of Cardiology).

factor 4 (PF4), although it may also occur with LMWH. IgG or IgM antibodies bind to heparin-PF4 complexes and activate platelets through their Fc receptor, causing platelet consumption and the development of microthrombi, leading to extension of previous thrombosis or a recurrent event. HIT (heparin-induced thrombocytopenia) should be suspected in any patient on UFH, or with previous exposure to heparin, whose platelet count falls by >30% within 4–10 days of exposure to heparin, especially if there is evidence of disseminated intravascular coagulation, systemic allergy or new thrombosis. A validated scoring system can be used to calculate the likelihood of HIT and determine the need for further investigation and management. As these patients are highly prothrombotic, therapeutic anticoagulation with an alternative anticoagulant must be initiated. Options include danaparoid, fondaparinux and argatroban, while further use of heparin is contraindicated.

Osteoporosis
The risk is primarily associated with long-term use of heparin (>6 months). It occurs because of heparin binding to osteoblasts causing releases of factors that activate osteoclasts.

Bleeding
Anticoagulation inevitably increases the risk of bleeding events. The annual incidence of bleeding requiring hospital admission for patients on warfarin is approximately 4.3%. Measures to reverse anticoagulation are therefore important, as well as general haemostatic measures, including applied pressure, surgical management and potential use of anti-fibrinolytic agents such as tranexamic acid.

Reversal of anticoagulation

Heparin

The action of heparin is antagonised by protamine sulphate, which forms an inactive complex with the drug. One milligram of protamine given intravenously reverses approximately 80–100 iu of UFH if given within 15 min of exposure. The effect on LMWH is incomplete. Caution must be taken in those patients with a fish allergy, as protamine is extracted from fish roe and sensitivity may occur.

Warfarin

Vitamin K can be given either orally or intravenously, with the route determined by the degree and speed at which reversal is required. However, there are certain circumstances where life- or limb-threatening bleeding means that complete reversal of warfarin is required more quickly. This can be achieved with prothrombin complex concentrate (PCC), containing factors II, VII, IX and X. In addition, erratic INR control may not always present with bleeding, but these patients are at a higher risk of complications. Box 15.3 shows measures to reverse warfarin. It is notable that patients in whom the INR is within the target therapeutic range less than 58% of the time are more at harm from being on warfarin than they would be without it.

Box 15.3 **Measures to reverse warfarin**

Measures to reverse warfarin

- Asymptomatic over-anticoagulation
  - Patients with an international normalized ratio (INR) >5.0 who are not bleeding should have 1–2 doses of warfarin withheld. The cause of the elevated INR should be investigated and the maintenance dose may need to be reduced.
  - Patients with an INR of ≥8·0 who are not bleeding should receive 1–5 mg of oral vitamin K. The INR should be rechecked the following day in case an additional dose of vitamin K is required.
- Bleeding
  - Patients with non-major bleeding should receive 1–3 mg of intravenous vitamin K.
  - Patients with major bleeding should be given 25–50 U/kg of PCC and 5 mg of intravenous vitamin K (1B).
  - Fresh frozen plasma produces suboptimal anticoagulation reversal but can be used if PCC is not available.
  - Recombinant factor VIIa is not recommended for emergency anticoagulation reversal.
  - All hospitals managing patients on warfarin should stock PCC containing factors II, VII, IX and X.

- Reversal for surgery
  - If possible delay surgery for 6–12 h to allow correction with intravenous vitamin K.
  - For emergency surgery that cannot be delayed, reverse with PCC and intravenous vitamin K.

NOACs

There is currently no available antidote for any of the new oral anticoagulants. In the event of major bleeding or emergency surgery, reversal of the anticoagulation effect can be difficult. Current guidelines suggest the use of tranexamic acid and PCC or activated prothrombin complex concentrate (aPCC, i.e. FEIBA) but there is little evidence regarding this at present and work is ongoing in this area.

Further reading

Baglin T, Barrowcliffe TW, Cohen A and Greaves M. The British Committee for Standards in Haematology: guidelines on the use and monitoring of heparin. *Br J Haematol* 2006a;**133**:19–34.

Baglin TP, Brush J and Streiff M. The British Committee for Standards in Haematology: guidelines on use of vena cava filters. *Br J Haematol* 2006b;**134**:590–595.

Baglin T, Keeling D and Kitchen S. Effects on routine coagulation screens and assessment of anticoagulant intensity in patients taking oral dabigatran or rivaroxaban: guidance from the British Committee for Standards in haematology. *Br J Haematol* 2012;**159**:427–429.

Guyatt GH, Akl EA, Crowther M, *et al.* Antithrombotic therapy and prevention of thrombosis, 9th edition: American College of chest physicians evidence-based clinical practice guidelines. *Chest* 2012;**141**:2S–6S.

Keeling D, Baglin T, Tait C, *et al.* Guidelines on oral anticoagulation with warfarin: guidance from the British Committee for Standards in Haematology. *Br J Haematol* 2011;**154**:311–324.

Makris M, Van Veen J, Tait C, *et al.* Guideline on the management of bleeding in patients on antithrombotic agents. *Br J Haematol* 2013;**160**:35–46.

Palareti G, Leali N, Coccheri S, *et al.* Bleeding complications of oral anticoagulant treatment: an inception-cohort, prospective collaborative study (ISCOAT). *Lancet* 1996;**348**:423–428.

Stansby G, Agarwal R, Ballard S, *et al.* NICE clinical guideline, CG144, venous thromboembolic diseases: the management of venous thromboembolic diseases and the role of thrombophilia testing. *NICE* 2012.

Treasure T, Carter K, Gautam N, *et al.* NICE Clinical guidelines, CG92. Reducing the risk of venous thromboembolism (deep vein thrombosis and pulmonary embolism) in patients admitted to hospital. *NICE* 2011.

Tosetto A, Iorio A, Marcucci M, *et al.* Predicting disease recurrence in patients with previous unprovoked venous thromboembolism: A proposed prediction score (DASH). *J Thromb Haemost.* 2012;**366**:1019–1025.

Turpie AGG, Chin BSP and Lip GYH. Venous thromboembolism: treatment strategies. *BMJ* 2002;**325**(7370):948.

Index

ABC of Arterial and Venous Disease, Third Edition.
Edited by Tim England and Akhtar Nasim.
© 2015 John Wiley & Sons, Ltd. Published 2015 by John Wiley & Sons, Ltd.

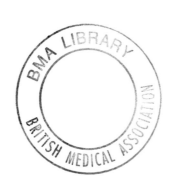

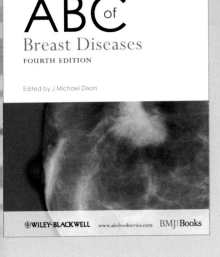

ABC of Breast Diseases

4TH EDITION

J. Michael Dixon
Western General Hospital, Edinburgh, UK

Breast diseases are common and often encountered by health professionals in primary care. While the incidence of breast cancer is increasing, earlier detection and improved treatments are helping to reduce breast cancer mortality. The *ABC of Breast Diseases, 4th Edition*:

- Provides comprehensive guidance to the assessment of symptoms, how to manage common breast conditions and guidelines on referral
- Covers congenital problems, breast infection and mastalgia, before addressing the epidemiology, prevention, screening and diagnosis of breast cancer and outlines the treatment and management options for breast cancer within different groups
- Includes new chapters on the genetics, prevention, management of high risk women and the psychological aspects of breast diseases
- Is ideal for GPs, family physicians, practice nurses and breast care nurses as well as for surgeons and oncologists both in training and recently qualified as well as medical students

AUGUST 2012 | 9781444337969 | 168 PAGES | £27.99/US$46.95/€35.90/AU$52.95

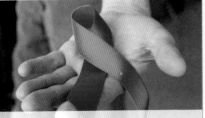

ABC of HIV and AIDS

6TH EDITION

Michael W. Adler, Simon G. Edwards, Robert F. Miller,
Gulshan Sethi & Ian Williams
University College London Medical School; Mortimer Market Centre, London; University College London; St Thomas' Hospital, London Medical School; University College London Medical School

Since the previous edition, big advances have been made in treatment, knowledge of the disease and epidemiology. The problem of AIDS in developing countries has become a major political and humanitarian issue.

- Edited by the Director of the Department for Sexually Transmitted Diseases, *ABC of HIV and AIDS, 6th Edition* is an authoritative guide to the epidemiology, incidence, and most up to date management of HIV and AIDS
- Reflects the constantly changing knowledge of the disease and its manifestations, new developments in drug and non-drug management, sociological and political issues
- Includes 6 new chapters on conditions associated with AIDS and further concentration on the community effects of the disease, and the situation of women with AIDS
- Ideal for all levels of health care workers caring for HIV and AIDS patients

JUNE 2012 | 9781405157001 | 144 PAGES | £24.99/US$49.95/€32.90/AU$47.95

ABC of Pain

Lesley A. Colvin & Marie Fallon
Western General Hospital, Edinburgh; University of Edinburgh

Pain is a common presentation and this brand new title focuses on the pain management issues most often encountered in primary care. *ABC of Pain*:

- Covers all the chronic pain presentations in primary care right through to tertiary and palliative care and includes guidance on pain management in special groups such as pregnancy, children, the elderly and the terminally ill
- Includes new findings on the effectiveness of interventions and the progression to acute pain and appropriate pharmacological management
- Features pain assessment, epidemiology and the evidence base in a truly comprehensive reference
- Provides a global perspective with an international list of expert contributors

JUNE 2012 | 9781405176217 | 128 PAGES | £24.99/US$44.95/€32.90/AU$47.95

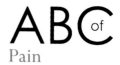
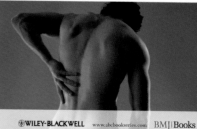
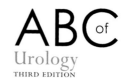

ABC of Urology

3RD EDITION

Chris Dawson & Janine Nethercliffe
Fitzwilliam Hospital, Peterborough; Edith Cavell Hospital, Peterborough

Urological conditions are common, accounting for up to one third of all surgical admissions to hospital. Outside of hospital care urological problems are a common reason for patients needing to see their GP.

- *ABC of Urology, 3rd Edition* provides a comprehensive overview of urology
- Focuses on the diagnosis and management of the most common urological conditions
- Features 4 additional chapters: improved coverage of renal and testis cancer in separate chapters and new chapters on management of haematuria, laparoscopy, trauma and new urological advances
- Ideal for GPs and trainee GPs, and is useful for junior doctors undergoing surgical training, while medical students and nurses undertaking a urological placement as part of their training programme will find this edition indispensable

MARCH 2012 | 9780470657171 | 88 PAGES | £23.99/US$37.95/€30.90/AU$47.95

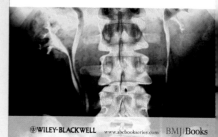

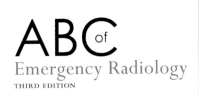

ABC of Emergency Radiology
3RD EDITION

Otto Chan
London Independent Hospital

The *ABC of Emergency Radiology, 3rd Edition* an invaluable resource for accident and emergency staff, trainee radiologists, medical students, nurses, radiographers and all medical personnel involved in the immediate care of trauma patients.

- Follows a systematic approach to assessing radiographs
- Each chapter covers a different part of the body, leading through the anatomy for ease of use
- Includes clear explanations and instructions on the appearances of radiological abnormalities with comparison to normal radiographs throughout
- Incorporates over 400 radiographs

JANUARY 2013 | 9780470670934 | 144 PAGES | £29.99/US$48.95/€38.90/AU$57.95

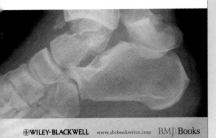

ABC of Resuscitation
6TH EDITION

Jasmeet Soar, Gavin D. Perkins & Jerry Nolan
Southmead Hospital, Bristol; University of Warwick, Coventry; Royal United Hospital, Bath

A practical guide to the latest resuscitation advice for the non-specialist *ABC of Resuscitation, 6th Edition*:

- Covers the core knowledge on the management of patients with cardiopulmonary arrest
- Includes the 2010 European Resuscitation Council Guidelines for Resuscitation
- Edited by specialists responsible for producing the European and UK 2010 resuscitation guidelines

DECEMBER 2012 | 9780470672594| 144 PAGES | £28.99/US$47.95/€37.90/AU$54.95

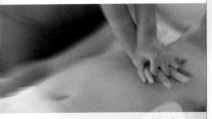

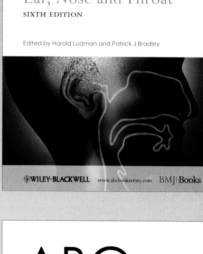
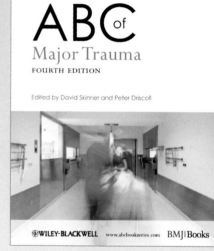
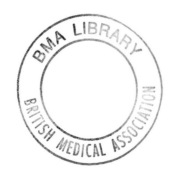

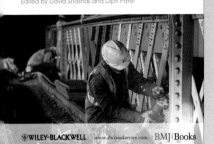

ABC of Occupational and Environmental Medicine

3RD EDITION

David Snashall & Dipti Patel
Guy's & St. Thomas' Hospital, London; Medical Advisory Service for Travellers Abroad (MASTA)

Since the publication of last edition, there have been huge changes in the world of occupational health. It has become firmly a part of international public health, and in Britain there is now a National Director for Work and Health. This fully updated new edition embraces these changes and:

- Provides comprehensive guidance on current occupational and environmental health practice and legislation
- Concentrates on the newer kinds of occupational disease, for example 'RSI', pesticide poisoning and electromagnetic radiation, where exposure and effects are difficult to understand
- Places an emphasis on work, health and well-being, and the public health benefits of work, the value of work, disabled people at work, the aging workforce, and vocational rehabilitation
- Includes chapters on the health effects of climate change and of occupational health and safety in relation to migration and terrorism

NOVEMBER 2012 | 9781444338171 | 168 PAGES | £27.99/US$44.95/€38.90/AU$52.95

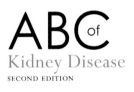

ABC of Kidney Disease

2ND EDITION

David Goldsmith, Satish Jayawardene & Penny Ackland
Guy's & St. Thomas' Hospital, London; King's College Hospital, London; Melbourne Grove Medical Practice, London

Nephrology is sometimes considered a complicated and specialized topic and the illustrative ABC format will help GPs quickly and easily assimilate the information needed. *ABC of Kidney Disease, 2nd Edition*:

- Is a practical guide to the most common renal diseases to enable non-renal health care workers to screen, identify, treat and refer renal patients appropriately and to provide the best possible care
- Covers organizational aspects of renal disease management, dialysis and transplantation
- Provides an explanatory glossary of renal terms, guidance on anaemia management and information on drug prescribing and interactions
- Has been fully revised in accordance with new guidelines

OCTOBER 2012 | 9780470672044 | 112 PAGES | £27.99/US$44.95/€35.90/AU$52.95

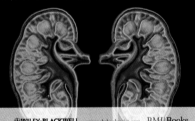